Women,
Health,
and Culture

A **Health Care for Women International** Publication

Carole Ann McKenzie, CNM, PhD
and **Phyllis Noerager Stern,** DNS, RN, FAAN, *Editors*

Women,
Health,
and Culture

Edited by

Phyllis Noerager Stern
School of Nursing
Dalhousie University
Halifax, Nova Scotia, Canada

2/04
● HEMISPHERE PUBLISHING CORPORATION
Washington   New York   London

DISTRIBUTION OUTSIDE THE UNITED STATES
McGRAW–HILL INTERNATIONAL BOOK COMPANY
Auckland   Bogotá   Guatemala   Hamburg   Johannesburg   Lisbon
London   Madrid   Mexico   Montreal   New Delhi   Panama   Paris
San Juan   São Paulo   Singapore   Sydney   Tokyo   Toronto

I dedicate this book to my family and my other mentors; especially to my husband Milt, the original Gray Gorilla, to my son Roger who is always there for me, and to my daughter Paula who thinks I can do it all.

I also dedicate the book to my mother Grace Ann Zoellen Noerager, who was a woman of great courage, and to my father Phillip Julius Noerager who was a man of rare wisdom. You were right, Pop, you can't expect 100 percent.

WOMEN, HEALTH, AND CULTURE

1 2 3 4 5 6 7 8 9 0   B R B R   8 9 8 7 6 5

This book was set in Press Roman by Hemisphere Publishing Corporation. The editors were Christine Flint, Amy Whitmer, and Marybeth Janney; the production supervisor was Miriam Gonzalez; and the typesetter was Peggy Rote.
Braun-Brumfield, Inc. was printer and binder.

Library of Congress Cataloging in Publication Data
Main entry under title:

Women, health, and culture.

(Health care for women international)
Includes bibliographies and index.
1. Women—Health and hygiene—Cross-cultural studies.   2. Health behavior—Cross-cultural studies. 3. Decision-making—Cross-cultural studies.   I. Stern, Phyllis Noerager.   II. Series.   [DNLM: 1. Cross-Cultural Comparison.   2. Health.   3. Women.   WA 300 W8725] RA564.85.W658   1985   362.1'042'088042   85-5533 ISBN 0-89116-372-7

CONTENTS

CONTRIBUTORS

L. MARIE ALLEN, EdD, RN
Professor and Coordinator
Graduate Studies in Adult Nursing
College of Nursing
Northwestern State University
Shreveport, Louisiana

JOYCEEN S. BOYLE, PhD, RN
Associate Professor
College of Nursing
University of Utah
Salt Lake City, Utah

MARY ATCHITY CALHOUN, MS,
RN
Cardiovascular Patient Educator
St. Elizabeth Hospital
Beaumont, Texas

MARY EVE BASKERVILLE
COUSINS, MSN, RN
Utilization Review Coordinator
SIGNA Healthplan of Shreveport/
Bossier City
Shreveport, Louisiana

PHYLLIS B. GRAVES, DSN, RN
Professor and Department Head
Bachelor of Science Program
College of Nursing
Northwestern State University
Shreveport, Louisiana

CHANDICE C. HARRIS, MS, RN
Doctoral Student
School of Nursing
University of Michigan
Ann Arbor, Michigan

ELEANOR KRASSEN MAXWELL,
PhD
County Planner
Kern County Economic Opportunities
Corporation
Bakersfield, California

SUE HOLLAND PYLES, MSN, RN
Assistant Professor
Division of Nursing
College of Life Sciences
Louisiana Tech University
Ruston, Louisiana

MARY DELL SHELTON SCOTT,
MSN, RN
Instructor
School of Nursing
Southern Arkansas University
Magnolia, Arkansas

PHYLLIS NOERAGER STERN, DNS,
RN, FAAN
Professor and Director
School of Nursing
Dalhousie University
Halifax, Nova Scotia, Canada

VIRGINIA PETERSON TILDEN,
DNS, RN
Associate Professor
Mental Health Nursing
Oregon Health Sciences University
Portland, Oregon

ELIZABETH S. WOODWARD, PhD,
RN
Professor and Coordinator
Graduate Studies in Mental Health-
Psychiatric Nursing
College of Nursing
Northwestern State University
Shreveport, Louisiana

Professional nursing is both art and science. The clinical act of nursing practice is that special time when art and science come together to satisfy a patient or client's unique need. The objectivity of science merges with the subjectivity of art as the nurse personalizes the care to be given. Science principles and theories may be the same for all patients with a given nursing diagnosis, but the artistic application of principles and theories depends upon the unique individual with whom the nurse is working. Science is predictable and reliable; human behavior is not. Reactions to the conditions and circumstances surrounding health problems are dependent upon many social, economic, and cultural variables. Emotions, feelings, and deeply held values influence one's reactions to health problems and to the treatment prescribed for those problems. As nurse and patient interact, two cultural belief systems come face to face, for the caregiver's perspective may be quite different from the patient's. The skilled professional nurse will enter into the clinical act of nursing with sensitivity and knowledge that combines the art and science of our profession.

The chapters nestled between the covers of *Women, Health, and Culture* offer the reader face-to-face confrontations with values of selected cultural groups. The case study approach is used in part to focus our attention on the perceptions of groups of women in specific locations. In other chapters the systematic data collection and data analysis methodology of "grounded theory" are used to develop hypotheses related to cultural difference. The editor develops the concept of "cultural reasoning" by linking together the cultural environment from which patients come and the beliefs they hold.

Since health professionals have their own "cultural reasoning" the potential exists for nurses and other caregivers to impose their values upon an unwilling or misunderstood patient. The authors of the collected studies in this book describe, analyze, and hypothesize "cultural deafness" and "cultural blindness." If professionals cannot hear or see the beliefs, values, and emotions that surround the circumstances of health problems, they cannot be effective. This book suggests ways and means of providing "culturally sensitive" care.

In addition to the obvious contributions this book makes to the study of transcultural nursing and to grounded theory research, it makes a significant contribution to the growing body of literature about women and health. It is well recognized that women's health care needs have received more attention in recent times. Despite the recognition, however, there is comparatively little research to validate insights and intuition related to health needs of women, whose roles and responsibilities have markedly changed. Dr. Stern's book is about women. It opens a window and invites the reader to see and eventually to know women in the context of their cultural groups.

Shirley S. Chater
Council Associate
American Council on Education

PREFACE

Women have guarded the health of their families since the dawn of human time. Throughout the ages, women have tended the sick using special knowledge received from older women. Women's actions as guardians of health and healers of the sick have been guided by the beliefs of the cultural world in which they lived, and in which they live. For example, the pregnant woman in Berkeley who spent her early years in an eastern European ghetto of Chicago may pledge allegiance to the California health culture in which she wants to remain by jogging daily throughout gestation. She would then be casting off one of the cultural prescriptions of her upbringing, that of inactivity during pregnancy, and taking on a new western cultural prescription that espouses exercise during pregnancy. Both prescriptions are rooted in cultural values and both potentiate a healthy outcome.

The responsibility inherent in this work of women seems almost overwhelming: It is their job to oversee the health of the family, but if they try something new, move beyond the dictates of their culture, they find themselves on dangerous ground. If the something does not work, they run the risk of degradation and despair. We heap guilt on the woman who dares defy the cultural norms when she is in search of health or cure for her family. Sometimes we remove her from her kin if we perceive her transgressions to be of sufficient gravity. Is it any wonder then that most women keep to the safe path and obey the cultural norms that they have been taught? This volume is about women and the safe paths to health that they believe in.

I started writing about women and their safe paths to health when those paths seemed foreign to my own directions to safety. I wanted to understand what those women thought would help, and why. Women taught me a great deal about their health beliefs, and about their cultural reasons for doing things. I have learned enough that instead of feeling simply uninformed, I now know that I am enormously ignorant. But I try to learn: I listen, I ask questions when I can, and I observe.

Throughout this book a number of settings are described in which cultural environment contributes to fairly fixed values about health care. I call this point of view *cultural reasoning*, a way of health conceptualization and decision making based on values gained in particular cultural or ethnic environments.

Health professionals have their own cultural reasoning through which they make health-related decisions. The cultural reasoning of professionals is a mix of retained values from the culture of origin that are influenced by the values of professional cultural reasoning.

Professional values become superimposed on original values. Professionals believe, for example, that they know what is best for a client, and they believe that the client should comply with prescriptions derived from professional cultural reasoning.

Cultural reasoning becomes a foundation for resolution when professional and lay cultural prescriptions represent conflicting messages. In our collective research, we discovered that the values of cultural reasoning, lay or professional, are often so ingrained that when client and professional interact, they develop *cultural deafness,* that is, they cannot understand the meaning of what the other is saying. They also may suffer *cultural blindness;* they cannot see clinical data or the advantages of professional advice. This leads to a kind of psychosensory inertia reflecting cultural distortion wherein all information received takes on the cast of what they already know is right. Ultimately, the woman of a particular lay culture tries to follow her "right way," while the professional brands that woman noncompliant, and neither understands why the other is acting that way.

We believe this book offers the reader a conceptual model that incorporates concepts in cultural reasoning with health care for women. The first chapter deals with grounded theory, the research methodology used throughout most of the studies presented here to study culture. Although the grounded theory method is not the only one used by the contributors to this book, there has in recent years been a growing interest in clear usable descriptions of this investigative style. We believe that the one presented here is the most understandable to date.

Using the cultural decision-making model in Chapter 2 as a guide, the reader will be introduced to new ways of providing culturally sensitive care for clients. In this chapter, the difficulty parents have in deciding whether to circumcise their newborn is considered. As the author, Harris, says, "it's such a little thing" that as caregivers, we often overlook the perplexity of cultural values in this type of decision making.

Chapter 3 offers an example of how northern Louisiana black women make decisions regarding whose health care advice to seek and accept. The authors, Scott and Stern, suggest that the Ethno-Market Theory may apply to other ethnic and cultural groups as well.

Various chapters in this book address cultural reasoning in Caucasian and non-Caucasian populations. There are examples from Pilipino immigrants, Vietnamese immigrants, women of Guatemala, black women in the southern United States, and Caucasian women of the West Coast and the South. In Chapter 4, Calhoun describes some common beliefs of Vietnamese women that help us understand the cultural reasoning of this prevalent immigrant group. In Chapter 5, Boyle explains how the position of women in the society of a Guatemalan colonia influences self-care and the care given them. Examples are given in Chapter 6 of what constitutes the perception of abnormal behavior according to southern female black fundamentalists compared to perceptions of mental health professionals.

The culturally induced stress of childbearing in Pilipino-American families is the focus of Chapter 7, and provides a substantial work for the development of Stern's theory on the religiosity of care, which is presented in Chapter 8.

The culture shock of relocation that is experienced by caregivers is explored in Chapter 9. The changes brought about by relocation were once thought to have a more significant impact on men. However, as more women realize that they too must move on to move up, the implications of these changes to the mental health of women and their families becomes a significant area of study.

The self-care evaluation tool presented in Chapter 10 seeks to preserve client self-direction while incorporating professional input. The case study that follows in Chapter 11 is a case in point that illustrates the counter-productive outcome that occurs when a caregiver as client becomes a victim of the cultural reasoning of her obstetrician and midwives.

Chapter 12 speaks to those of us who are specifically involved in teaching transcultural nursing. Although the strategies for heightening student awareness are designed for use on a basic level, this content brings us full circle to the value system of transcultural nursing itself.

The contributions of nurse colleagues in this book represent a diverse collection of individual culturally based studies. Although the book's primary focus is nursing, we hope that our colleagues in related disciplines will find this material pertinent to the care and teaching offered to female clients.

Other nurses who, like me, had to do something to get to the other side of their ignorance about women's cultural health beliefs wrote this volume with me. Their work may help you look at your own cultural beliefs about health as you compare them with people who hold beliefs at odds with your own. If you begin to wonder how important your own beliefs are, and if it is always necessary to impose them on your clients, then the purpose of these writings will be served.

I am deeply indebted to the authors who contributed to this book. The richness of their work speaks for itself. I am eternally grateful as well to the mentors and protégées who have influenced my life and my work.

Mary Eve Baskerville Cousins edited this work. Of the many typists who struggled through the several drafts of the manuscript, special mention is due Ms. Loretta Ware and Ms. Loreen Gilby.

Phyllis Noerager Stern

USING GROUNDED THEORY METHODOLOGY TO STUDY WOMEN'S CULTURALLY BASED DECISIONS ABOUT HEALTH

Phyllis Noerager Stern, DNS, RN, FAAN
Dalhousie University, Halifax, Nova Scotia

Sue Holland Pyles, RN, MSN
Louisiana Tech University, Ruston, Louisiana

A study of a culture implies a comparison with other cultures. The constant comparative processes that guide grounded theory methodology are ideal for defining cultural concepts generated through examination of the data.

Every creative act involves . . . a new innocence of perception, liberated from the cataract of accepted belief (Koestler, 1959).

When you return from a journey to a place that is foreign by the standards of home and describe what you have seen to your friends, you may find their attention span disappointingly short. As nurse researchers and educators interested in the development and use of cultural reasoning in cross-cultural nursing, we pondered the reason for this reaction in our colleagues, and concluded that *description alone is not enough.*

While description can provide factual accounts of phenomena identified within a culture, it is insufficient in expanding nursing knowledge because facts alone do not explain the underlying processes of those phenomena. Nursing is a practice discipline whose essence lies in processes. As such, nurses need more than descriptions. They want to know how, when, and where phenomena occur so that they can better understand, predict, and control situations. Furthermore, our colleagues are simply too busy, their minds are too cluttered with the business of living and dealing with the here-and-now, or their perception is too clouded by the cataract of accepted belief to be able to grasp the reality of a people, a culture, or a country in detail.

If our aim is to make the reality of other cultures known, if it is to assist our colleagues in achieving a new innocence of perception so that they can be more creative in their approaches to cultural issues, then we must move from description to explanation. To make the foreign familiar, our colleagues need conceptual pictures that explain the human condition elsewhere, so that they can compare it with their own human condition, in order to better understand the universals applicable to a variety of societies.

One universal of human behavior is that people compare phenomena in order to generate general rules. These rules, or principles of behavior, guide our actions until further study and collection of phenomena provides evidence that our hypotheses, or facts, are incorrect or need to be modified. "Oh," we say, "I see, it works in this situation, or context, but not in that." Through constant comparison of phenomena or data, with a fact or variable generated in the past, we learn to define the limits of the variable and its properties. For example, a Philippine-born woman may learn that to be polite, one defers to persons in authority. When she moves to the United States, this woman may find her ideas about courtesy no longer work. She may discover, as one woman living in Galveston, Texas, told us, "After we're here for a while, we learn that it's okay to be just as rude as the Americans." She had learned to define new limits for the variable *politeness,* and identified some of its properties: what is considered polite in the Philippines, does not necessarily hold true in the United States.

A study of culture implies a comparison with other cultures. One looks at another culture in order to find out its similarities and differences with one's own. That is to say, we check the new cultural norms against the facts of our own culture. If we want to compare cultures, the constant comparative processes that guide the grounded theory approach developed by Glaser and Strauss (1967) are ideal for defining concepts generated through examination of the data. For example, these processes were used in defining the variable *politeness* as it applies to various cultures (or contexts). As we compare phenomena with what we may have thought of as fact, we may hit upon a new hypothesis that links human behavior, or that accounts for a previously unknown limit to a given variable. As Maxwell and Maxwell (1980) so aptly put it,

> When we do research, we only know that we have discovered something new because we know that it doesn't fit or cannot be explained by our previous principles for explaining our experiences (p. 221).

Maxwell and Maxwell go on to point out that the human mind constantly processes information in a way that on a larger scale is known as research. We all use inductive processes, comparing specific phenomena to arrive at a general principle, and deductive processes, comparing phenomena with fact to derive specific conclusions or to discover unknown truths. Grounded theory methodology involves the use of inductive and deductive processes similar to the workings of the human mind as we attempt to understand it all.

Far from a simple puzzling over life, however, grounded theory methodology has formal rules of procedure, which if followed produce a substantive theory or conceptual definition of reality that is inherently valid, easily verifiable, and immediately applicable. In this chapter, we will discuss the value of using grounded theory in cultural studies, the method itself, and finally, the scope of its uses.

USING GROUNDED THEORY TO STUDY CULTURE

Grounded theory was developed as an analytical method to define reality in social situations. Prior to its development and the publication of *The Discovery of Grounded Theory: Strategies for Qualitative Research* by Glaser and Strauss in 1967, we were limited by the methodological approaches available to us in our attempts to capture the essence of cultures.

For one reason, the earlier and more traditionally accepted methods, such as experimental or quantitative survey design, do not have the potential for exploring and analyzing the multidimensional concepts and complexity of processes inherent in cross-cultural data. Clinton (1983) echoes this view in emphasizing the wide gap between theoretical advances and the methodological approaches used by investigators in studying the cultural dimensions of human experiences. Similarly, others have underscored the inadequacies of quantitative research in obtaining and interpreting all the knowledge that is potentially available about a particular phenomenon (Munhall, 1982; Oiler, 1982; Swanson & Chenitz, 1982).

In addition, the "preconceiving nature" (Glaser, 1978) of other methods in which hypotheses are derived from literature and then experimented upon, verified, and/or surveyed is restrictive. As Stern (1980) points out, it is impossible to test theory where no theory exists.

By its very nature, grounded theory is applicable to the study of cultures. The qualitative, holistic approach of grounded theory serves as a valuable heuristic in understanding and explaining human experience as it is lived, especially those subjective phenomena that can only be interpreted through the eyes of the beholder or those in which the whole is more than the sum of its parts. But perhaps the strongest case for the use of grounded theory is that it frees us "to discover what is going on, rather than assuming what should be going on" (Glaser, 1978, p. 159) in our attempts to understand fundamental processes and their applicability to problems and situations.

The crucial point remains in its practical application. In this section we present a few examples of the use of grounded theory to illustrate its applicability and value in studying culture.

Krassen-Maxwell (1979) used grounded theory to compare ethnographies of preindustrial societies. As far as we know, she pioneered the use of the method in this way. Maxwell looked at the meaning of ritual for such societies. What she found was a model-protegee system, where older models acted as mentors to young people so that the society's rituals could be carefully preserved. Maxwell's use of grounded theory demonstrates its applicability for discovering and understanding phenomena that are common to all societies.

On the other hand, grounded theory is helpful in exploring cultural differences. For instance, when Stern began working with Philippino-born clients and nurses in San Francisco, she was puzzled by the inefficacy of communication with these immigrants. Following the natural bent of the academic, she wanted to do a study about the problem. Stern did not know specific ethnographic rules for research, but because she had extensive experience in grounded theory methodology a study was put into motion. This study led to the discovery of grounded theory concerning barriers to health care that arise when cultural beliefs are different, as well as solutions used in crossing them (Stern, 1981, 1982a; Stern, Tilden, & Maxwell, 1980).

We do not suggest that Stern was the first investigator to use grounded theory to analyze cultural behavior, only that it is an atypical approach, the earlier and more familiar method being the ethnographic studies. Other examples of grounded theory cultural studies can be found in Lewis (1979), Louie (1975), O'Brien (1982), and Wadd (1983).

The way in which a grounded theory study goes beyond description to theoretical construct can be seen in Scott's study of the childbearing beliefs of northern Louisiana blacks (Scott, 1982a, 1982b; Scott & Stern, 1983).

Scott explained the processes and contexts that influenced decision-making about health care for these people. She developed a conceptual picture of the human condition that busy professionals can easily understand, one that is immediately applicable to their practice, and one that they may be able to apply to other ethnic groups as well. Professionals need such a picture because, as explained in our opening paragraph, *description alone would not have been enough!*

Another important advantage of the cultural study that defines concepts in a compact, dense, carefully integrated way is that the variables (concepts) described are readily and appropriately manageable for testing. Not only can nurses test these variables in practice, but nurse scientists have theories, grounded in data from nursing, that prove ripe for instrumentation (Cousins, 1981) and experimental studies. According to Glaser (1978), this is one of grounded theory's major functions.

To this point we have focused on the question, Why use grounded theory to study culture? But, enough convincing. As an Italian proverb states: "Between saying and doing there lies the ocean." This brings us to the next question: How is it done? For before grounded theory can be brought into the full realm of usefulness, its processes must be understood.

DEVELOPING A THEORY: RIGHT
AND LEFT BRAIN WORK

As we mentioned earlier, the processes used in the discovery of grounded theory are intricately related to the workings of the human mind. Grounded theory methodology is ideational and creative. The purpose of grounded theory is the development of theoretical constructs that explain the phenomenon under study. Generating grounded theory involves creative thinking in that the investigator must continuously analyze and synthesize the data as they are collected, coded, categorized, compared, and integrated into a well-fitting theory.

In the following discussion of these processes, we present the methodology as an orderly series of procedures. In truth, the methodology is anything but linear, and it certainly does not feel orderly when one is in the middle of it. As we move back and forth, from inductive to deductive modes, comparing phenomenon with phenomenon, phenomena with hypotheses, hypothesis with hypothesis, we use both the right and the left hemispheres of the brain.

> According to split brain theory, the right hemisphere of the brain is the seat of intuitive, holistic, spatial, simultaneous operations, such as creative imagining and philosophy. In contrast, the left hemisphere is concerned with linear sequential, and verbal operations—for example, reading and calculating (Demenses, 1980, p. 441).

The lateral, creative hemisphere of the brain recognizes the answer-behind-the-answer in interviews, reflects, on data, makes connections with other data and with the world outside the scene under study, and forms hypotheses. This is right brain or inductive activity. The left, or deductive, hemisphere gives stability and accuracy to the work with its recollection of facts, literature, and rules of procedure.

The techniques used in this type of theory development require a continual redesigning of the analysis, thereby allowing for the creative flow of ideas. Such creativity, according to Hartmann (1975) is a combination and association of facts, experience, and possibilities, and involves imagination and intuition. This synergy of logic and intuition pays off—two and two really do add up to five. Herein lies the conceptual transcending property of grounded theory. As data are conceptualized, the level of thought is elevated beyond what previously seemed distinct and incidental. Thus, grounded theory transcends previous descriptions and theories about an area by including and integrating other works as part of the data to be further compared to the emerging theory as an even more dense integrated theory of greater scope is generated (Glaser, 1978, p. 7).

Creativity and the production of new ideas requires a certain degree of psychic freedom, and, in particular, lateral thinking in which right hemisphere processes are used. Since right brain activity is holistic, it allows the analyst to see the wholes or overall patterns. Right brain thinking is characterized by intuition, imagination, and flashes of insight. Flashes of intuitive insight and creative breakthroughs almost always involve "recognition of patterns where there are gaps or literal differences" and/or "recognizing a known principle in disguise" (Blakeslee, 1980, p. 48). Koestler (1964) called this recognition of a disguised relationship "biosociation" because hidden relationships are found between two seemingly unrelated pieces of knowledge.

While the right brain has the ability to bridge gaps and make intuitive breakthroughs, creativity is equally dependent on the left brain's ability to verify them and convert them to the logical language of others. In grounded theory, we have an approach to theory development that allows us to use both the intuitive and the logical sides of our brains.

DEVELOPING A THEORY: THE ENTERPRISE

To accommodate our left brain, or reading hemisphere, we present the method in an orderly form. For the benefit of the right hemisphere, we offer a visual map of operations in the form of diagrams. These diagrams were developed and used by Pyles (1982a, 1982b, & 1983) to provide mental images of the abstract concepts and cyclic processes used in generating grounded theory, so that they could be "seen by the mind's eye" and be better understood.

As in previous writings (Stern, 1980; Stern, Allen, & Moxley, 1982), we use Maxwell and Maxwell's (1980) scheme for organizing the categories of procedure: (a) collection of empirical data, (b) concept formation, (c) concept development, (d) concept modification and integration, and (e) production of the research report. These processes produce a substantive theory, which emerges from and is supported by the data obtained. It is important to remember that these procedures are not done in linear steps. Rather, data collection and analysis occur simultaneously and systematically. Figure 1 shows the matrix nature of the method in which several processes are in operation at once.

Collection of Empirical Data

"Data for a grounded theory study may be collected from interview, observation, or documents, or from a combination of these sources" (Stern, Allen, & Moxley, 1982, p. 206). For example, in the

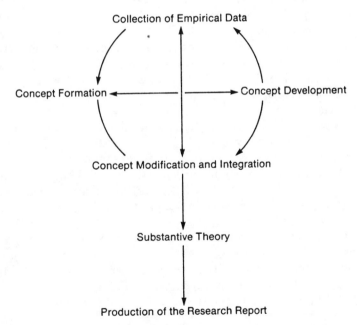

Figure 1. Processes of Grounded Theory Methodology. Processes in the method are lateral rather than linear as shown by the circular and connecting arrows.

Pilipino[*] study, data came from (a) over 400 hours of observation, (b) 246 interviews, (c) ethnographies, and (d) the reaction of audiences to whom the research was presented. This multifaceted approach to data collection is appropriate since the aim of the study was to discover variables that transcend finite times, places, and people. In other words, processes were sought that are found in all cultures. The purpose of grounded theory is to discover and generate explanations for such processes by identifying their dimensions and characteristics and the conditions under which they occur and vary. Acquiring different "slices of data" (Glaser & Strauss, 1967, p. 66) is necessary in order to have "different vantage points from which to understand a category and to develop its properties" (Wilson, 1977, p. 107).

How data are to be collected and recorded depends on the researcher, the study design, and the way in which those involved present their experiences. We will next describe the sources of data collection and some recording techniques.

Observation

Most studies start with observation—either participant observation, where you notice a problem in the practice area and decide to find out more about it, or looking about to see where the action is as you start a new area of study. These are called initial observations, and are quite appropriate to include with your other study data. No one comes to a study as a tabula rasa, and what you have previously observed, what you know, is important to the validity of the findings.

Observations may be guided by the familiar analytical scheme that asks for who, when, how, and why. But these soon give way to interactive research questions used in theoretical sampling (Denzin, 1970; Glaser & Strauss, 1967) concerning processes: What is going on? What are its properties? Under what conditions and with what consequences does it work? How did it come to be? What is it becoming? What does it mean?

Field notes are often used to record data and include the researcher's observations of an ongoing situation and reactions to the experiences shared with others in the field (Oiler, 1982; Stern, 1980). The questions which guide observations and the use of field notes to record the data obtained can also be used in interviewing.

---

[*]Tagalog, the national language of the Philippine Islands contains no "F" sound. Therefore the spelling Pilipino is more ethnosensitive than the more common Filipino.

Interviewing

New investigators tend to be nervous during their first interviews, so it may be helpful to have a guide with you to help you along. The interview guide might include instructions or reminders to give the subject a code name or to ask for certain demographic data, as well as open-ended questions that focus on the problem or area of interest. As the study proceeds, and hypotheses are formed, you can change or supplement these questions to clarify information or you can drop false leads to zero in on the pertinent data. Not all interviews are the same, just as people are not the same. Maintaining the individual uniqueness of subjects and the way they interpret their own personal experiences is one of the many ways you know your study is valid (Munhall, 1982).

In addition to an interview guide, a tape recorder is also helpful for storing data to new as well as seasoned investigators. For example, Pyles (1981) recorded her interviews with subjects to prevent any interference note taking might have on eye contact and the flow of ideas during the interviews, and to avoid the possibility of missing data that might later be considered significant. These goals were achieved, but we would be remiss in not showing you the other side of the coin. Interviews that lasted no more than 30 minutes took 4–8 hours to transcribe, and ranged from 20–40 double-spaced, typed pages. The important thing to remember is to allow time to transcribe the tapes, or make arrangements for a competent secretary to do it for you.

At first you may have trouble getting the information you want. Part of the problem may be that you have no clearly defined area of research. You explore. You learn interviewing techniques as you go along. Some examples may clarify interviewing vagaries.

In the Pilipino study, Stern began interviewing the nurses in the labor and delivery suite. Stern is a parent-child nurse, and she had already established rapport through her professional kinship. Pyles had a similar experience. When she began her study of the nursing culture in critical care (Pyles, 1981), she was able to establish relationships with those nurses because as a critical care nurse herself, she knew what they were talking about. On the other hand, when Scott began her interviews to find out the childbearing beliefs of northern Louisiana black women, the women told her almost nothing. Scott had thought that because she herself was a black woman, other black women would open up to her. After many painful, frustrating attempts at obtaining data, Scott realized that her interviewees saw her as a nurse, rather than a peer. Finally, Scott started her interviews by telling about some of the folk beliefs she held as a child and a young woman. Then she asked, "Has anyone in your family ever believed anything like that?" The data came pouring out.

Documents

Naturally you will want to review relevant literature as you begin the formal part of your study. For one thing, you want to know if someone has already answered the question that puzzles you. Also, existing concepts that have relevance for your study will help you understand your data, and can be used to support and develop new concepts. However, keep in mind that where you start in the literature may not be where the focus of your study leads you. For example, Pyles discovered that critical care nurses develop and use what she calls *nursing gestalt,* a combination of knowledge, identifying cues, categorization, differentiation, and gut feelings that emphasize the importance of both the conceptual process and the sensory act (Pyles & Stern, 1983). Nursing gestalt enables experienced nurses to forecast a patient's prognosis before the lab results or the monitors depict a change. This finding sent the investigator back to the library to find out what she could about gestalt theory.

Audience Reaction

As the research advances and hypotheses are formed, you begin presenting your ideas to colleagues and other audiences. A presentation of your findings usually offers an another opportunity for data collection as people give you additional examples. To be absolutely ethical, you should obtain permission to include the example with your study data.

In truth, a grounded theory is not finite. Even though you write the initial research report at some point, further communication developing into new insights can be included in subsequent publications. In addition what is discovered in one study may have relevance for a previous or future study. This point will be elaborated on in the discussion of the scope of grounded theory.

Concept Formation

Concepts in a grounded theory come from the data and are formed through an analytical process that begins at the time of data collection and continues throughout the investigation. As data are collected, coding and categorizing processes are used in generating a tentative conceptual framework.

Coding

In the initial analysis, a system of open coding is used whereby the data are examined line by line as the researcher seeks and identifies processes. As data are coded, key words or codes that symbolize an event or process are underscored and written in the margin of the field notes beside their indicators in the data. In this way, codes are pulled from the data and can be used in later analysis. These codes are called substantive codes because they name or describe the data from which they were derived. For example, when Pilipino women related that Western nurses shamed them, Stern (1981) labeled the remark "shaming."

Once coding begins, the researcher starts interpreting the data. Ideas or hunches can occur at any time or in any place, and if not recorded instantly, an important idea can be lost. A memo method that is used to capture these ideas will be discussed later.

Categorizing

Once data are coded, they seem to cluster together into naturally related categories. Just what is a category in the research sense? It is the same as any other category. One of the most common categorical schemes is arranging materials in alphabetical order. In this scheme drugs, references, friends' names, and the like are placed into alphabetical groups or categories because they seem to belong together. We tend to categorize people we meet in much the same way: by sex, race, beauty, culture, profession, intellectual ability, and age. In the Pilipino study, categories emerged that related to styles of address, problems with language, and learning new ways.

As interrelationships are identified among the categories, the researcher links them together to form a tentative conceptual framework. Figure 2 summarizes the processes used in concept formation.

Collaborating

One generally collects data solo. However, coding and categorizing go much better in a collaborative situation where a group of researchers review the data at the same time, and try to identify commonalities. It may be considered more suitable to write something that sounds orderly (to appeal to the left hemisphere) such as, "As data are received, the analyst applies a system of substantive codes, so called because they codify the substance of the data; they often use the very words used by the actors themselves" (Stern, Allen, & Moxley, 1982, p. 207). But the real life situation is something like

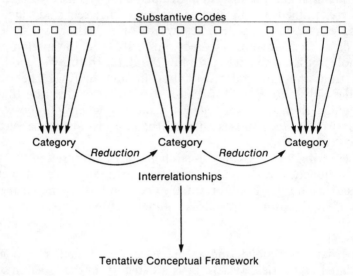

Figure 2. Concept Formation. Substantive codes, represented by the small boxes, group together to form categories. As the interrelationships between categories become clear, several can be reduced to form larger concepts as shown.

the following scenario. The actors are collaborative researchers reading the data from interviews with nurses:

> ... What's happening here—it seems like they're doing a lot of *delaying*.
> ... that, and there's a lot of talk about *time* ... see this on page 3.
> ... I learned to believe people when they say they're having pain.
> ... Use that, as one nurse said, "I learned to believe people ..."
> ... You know what? They're applying *objective data,* like time and when the patient had the surgery, to judge a *subjective* experience, pain!
> ... Let's get back to the data (Simulation of a coding session for Brocato's nursing culture study, "Right and Left Brain Nursing, Pain Assessment on an Orthopedic Ward," 1982).

It can be seen by the example above that developing a concept goes best in a collegial setting. This scenario also illustrates how all operations in the development of a theory go on simultaneously.

Concept Development

Once concepts are formed, three major steps are necessary to expand and densify the emerging theory: reduction, selective sampling of the literature, and selective sampling of the data. Through these processes, the core variable emerges as the central integrative category or theoretical scheme.

Reduction

During the analysis, many concepts or categories and their theoretical properties are generated as the investigator compares incident to incident and concept to incident to establish the underlying principle and its variations. Then, as category is compared with category, the analyst begins to understand how they relate to one another. At this point, one searches for a higher level category under which these categories may be subsumed, and in this way reduced. In the Pilipino study, a number of categories were reduced to fit under three higher-order categories: approach, custom, and language. For example, the categories of styles of address, pattenrs of nonconfrontation and indirect communication, and personal approach to social interactions were seen to be linked, as these actions all served to maintain the Filipinos' self-respect, and helped them avoid feelings of shame. Thus, these categories were reduced to the category of styles of approach and became its properties.

Reduction of categories to core variables, or theoretical codes, involves a more theoretical analysis than clustering coded data because core variables are major processes that explain rather than name or describe the phenomenon under study. For instance in Stern's study, approach, custom, and language earned their way into the theory because they offered the most complete explanation of how cultural barriers caused communication breakdown between Pilipinos and Western nurses.

Selective Sampling of the Literature

Once the emerging theory is sufficiently developed, the literature is carefully reviewed for concepts that are related to the theory. Through integration of ideas, the existing literature is used as supporting data for the emerging theory, and is woven into its matrix of data, category, and conceptualization. In other words, if concepts in the literature fit the emerging theory, use them to tell your story; if they are not relevant and do not really fit or work, leave them out. Otherwise, the data can be forced in the wrong direction. By the same token, if the literature is reviewed before the generated theory is sufficiently developed, preconceived concepts can lead you astray or contaminate your efforts to generate concepts from the data. This is not to say that a particularly good theory that has relevance for a study cannot be reviewed earlier. But when this is the case, the generated theory usually extends or transcends the extant theory, and therefore represents more than hypothesis verification or replication of previous study.

We hasten to caution the reader at this point that publication in a juried journal does not in and of itself make a piece of research valid, reliable, or useful. For example, the literature clearly points out that Pilipinos tend to be shy and deferent. We accepted that concept, in spite of data to the contrary. Fortunately, Pilipinos, who audienced our research, pointed out the error of our ways. Finally we were able to hear, as women like the Pilipino immigrant in Galveston told us, "After we're here a while, we find out it's okay to be just as rude as the Americans." So we learned that shyness and deference depend on length of stay. We did not find that in the literature.

Selective Sampling of Data

As the main concepts or core variables become apparent, additional data are collected in a selective manner to identify their properties and to develop and verify the emerging hypotheses. "I think this is what is happening," you say, but you are not sure your hypotheses are valid. You ask a few more people if what you perceive provides an accurate account of the situation: "It happens in this contest, under these conditions, with these consequences . . . What about that?" Selective sampling of data gives the answer.

Grounded theorists, like other researchers, go to a great deal of trouble to make sure their findings are accurate. As Glaser and Strauss (1967) tell us: selective sampling is used to find out the "truth"

> Thus facts are replicated with comparative evidence, either internally (within a study), externally (outside a study), or both. Sociologists generally agree that replications are the best means for validating facts (p. 23).

However, since a grounded theory study cannot be replicated by later studies, concepts must be verified as to their propriety for the emerging theory as the research advances. Therefore, hypotheses, generated from the data, are tested by collecting additional data that support or disprove their validity. Concepts that cannot be supported in this way are dropped. This process is deductive in nature because previously formed concepts are consequently verified.

Selective sampling of data also has an inductive aspect because it involves a search to identify the properties of the core variables and to develop the emerging hypotheses. Data are now collected to expand, limit, and dimensionalize the variables or concepts by their relevant properties, elements, or divisions. Saturation of a category is reached when no new information is obtained that further explains that particular aspect of the emerging hypothesis. Data collection then ceases for that category. The investigator must now determine the fit of the core variables in order to integrate them into a well constructed conceptual framework or substantive theory.

Emergence of the Core Variable

For some, the term "emerge" has magical and mystical connotations. However, core variables do not merely appear out of thin air. Rather, as we have tried to explain in the previous discussion, they are discovered as the investigator carefully and systematically uses the process of reduction and comparison. As with any new discovery, a certain degree of creativity is required and results in what Glaser (1978) calls "drugless highs." As you continuously analyze the data, comparing categories for their relationships and properties, and as you talk with your colleagues and subjects, suddenly (albeit out of pain and depression), you see the study holistically. A flash of insight tells you what the study is all about. Your left brain kept track of the facts, and your right brain brings it all together. Eureka! You have discovered the core variable.

A core variable simply means a central theme or concept that holds all the data together. In Pyles' study it was nursing gestalt; Stern's Pilipino study had covariables: communication breakdown, the obstacle to learning in cross cultural health teaching; and a co-variable, showing respect mutually which repairs the damage. While exciting and rewarding, there was certainly nothing magical about the "eureka" experiences involved in the discovery of these core variables. A great deal of time and effort preceded their illumination, and more went into verification.

To be credible, the core variables, or theory, must be well integrated, easy to understand, relevant to the empirical world, and must explain the major variation in the process or phenomena studied. The final test of credibility lies with the subject group. If a theory fits, the audience grasps the idea quickly, heads nod in agreement, eyes light up, and they say, "That's it. That's just the way it is!" Such responses provide evidence of a theory's acceptability, and give credence to the assumption that it presents an accurate reflection of reality.

In sum, the phase of concept development involves processes that result in the identification, conceptualization, and verification of core variables and their properties. These processes are illustrated in Figure 3. Properties are identified and their variations

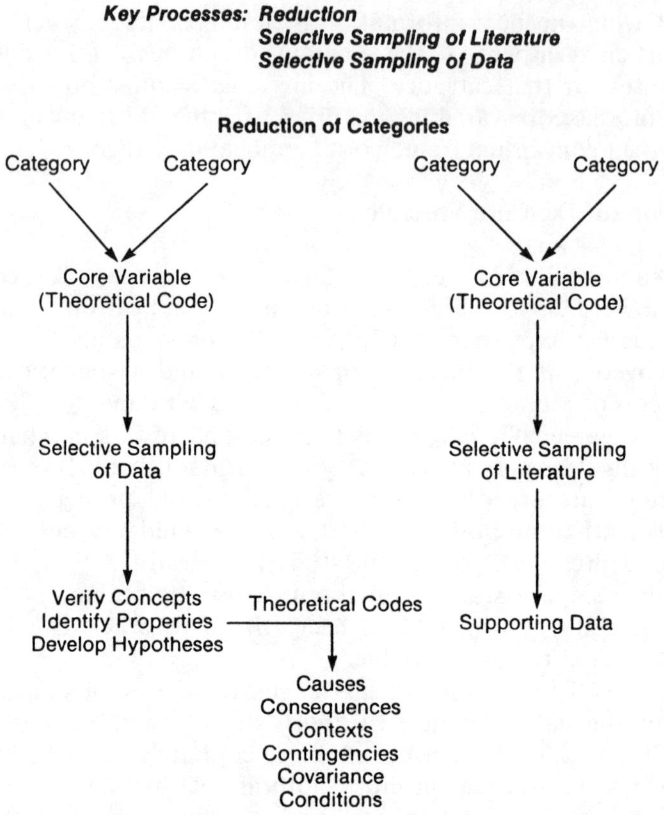

Key Processes: *Reduction*
Selective Sampling of Literature
Selective Sampling of Data

Reduction of Categories

Category   Category   Category   Category

Core Variable
(Theoretical Code)   Core Variable
(Theoretical Code)

Selective Sampling
of Data   Selective Sampling
of Literature

Verify Concepts   Theoretical Codes
Identify Properties ———————   Supporting Data
Develop Hypotheses

Causes
Consequences
Contexts
Contingencies
Covariance
Conditions

Figure 3. Concept Development. The researcher groups together data, categories, and literature and through the use of theoretical codes, brings out the conceptual meaning of the variable as seen at the bottom of this figure.

are explained by means of theoretical codes, as the lower part of the figure demonstrates.

Concept Modification and Integration

In order to present an integrated, well explained theory, the researcher uses the processes of theoretical coding and memoing. Through these processes, the emerging theory is modified, or delimited, to a smaller number of higher level concepts or core variables. Once again, the analyst compares concept with more highly developed concept to discover their theoretical relationships, and related concepts are compared with data for validation. Theoretical completeness is achieved as the core variables are expanded, dimensionalized, saturated, delimited, and integrated into a well constructed substantive theory. The processes used in concept modification and integration are depicted schematically in Figure 4. Although this phase is a culminating process, the matrix nature of continuous comparative analysis can be seen in that this phase overlaps and occurs in concert with the other phases.

Theoretical Coding

The process of theoretical coding is a way of relating variables theoretically to produce what Glaser and Strauss (1967) call a "dense" theoretical scheme. Without theoretical codes, the research ends up a simple description. Description is highly useful. However, as we pointed out earlier, description lacks the quality of a well defined concept. In theory development, it is not enough to describe the characteristics of a social phenomenon. As Artinien (1982) said, "Tentative theoretical statements can be made only when an attempt is made to link the causes and consequences of the variables

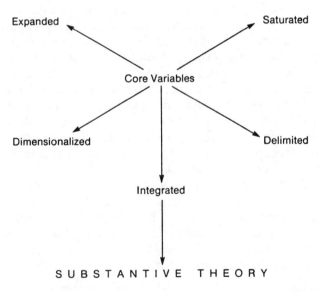

Figure 4. Concept Modification and Integration. The processes depicted here result in a well-defined concept. A carefully written description completes the work.

identified in the social phenomenon" (p. 379). Theoretical coding provides the analyst with a strategy for doing this.

Theoretical codes, applied to data and to categories, provide the opportunity to think about the data in theoretical ways. A conceptual definition is achieved as one considers a variable from the point of view of its causes, consequences, contexts, contingencies, covariances, and conditions. Glaser (1978) supplies several "families" of such codes that can be applied to the data to enhance their abstraction.

Memoing

Writing memos is a method of recording and preserving analytical ideas, hunches, abstractions, and emerging hypotheses as they occur. Remember that although the phases of grounded theory methodology have been presented in linear steps, they really occur simultaneously. Insights flash through your mind all the time and throughout the analysis. They occur in unlikely places and at any hour of the day or night. *Write them down as they occur!* Otherwise, you will lose them. For example, we began writing memos for this chapter months ago: "Description alone is not enough" was one of them.

Memos are conceptual elaborations of ideas about codes and categories and their relationships. While ideational, memos are sparked by the data, and in this way they are grounded. As data are collected and analyzed, memos can be jotted down in the margin of field notes near their indicators. However, as the study proceeds, the analyst's mind becomes steeped in the data, and an idea can strike at any time or in any place. These ideas are often captured on scraps of paper, and include a reference to the data that sparked them. Memos, with their indicators from the data, are then placed on typewritten pages or cards captioned with the relevant code or category. Any supporting data obtained through selective sampling of the literature or additional data collection is also included. Thus, memos contain the conceptual groundwork for generating theory.

Before the research report is written memos need to be categorized. This provides another opportunity to cluster concepts; to see how they integrate with one another. Memos are sorted into piles and then organized in such a way as to produce the best integration of the theory. Sorted memos provide the structure, content, and organization for the manuscript.

Production of the Research Report

The research report gives a clear, precise rendition of the theory substantiated by the data and the existing literature. Most first-time grounded theorists believe their theory so wholeheartedly that they assume their readers can guess what it has taken them months to discover. Conclusions must be explained in detail, including the range of data on which the analysis was made. Since data is where the theory originates, findings must be supported with data. Therefore, the style of the written report is an integration of theory, findings, and discussion.

SYSTEMATIC FORM AND ANALYSIS

Grounded theory method lends itself to a wide range of resources, from the personal biography, through connections with past study, to a meta-analysis of several studies. These resources comprise a variety of systematic ways in which data can be collected, organized, and interpreted.

Personal Biography

By personal biography, we mean either an elaborate case study spanning months or years with an in-depth analysis of processes, trajectories, and phases, or, as in the example we provide, a participant observation and analysis comparing two environments and the impact of change on an individual.

Example

When Stern made a major career and geographic move, she expected to feel a certain amount of culture shock living and working in Louisiana after living most of her life in the San Francisco Bay Area. But the culture shock was more profound than she expected. In an attempt to relieve the pain by intellctualizing the event, Stern kept careful field notes on her reactions, on time sequences (phases of shock), and on the comparative conditions that helped her overcome the shock. Later in the study, she asked colleagues, friends, and acquaintances about some of her impressions (selective sampling) and in this way validated her findings. Interestingly enough, the literature search was the last step in her collection of data; was her reaction typical? Stern found that it was typical considering theoretical codes of contexts, contingencies, and causes.

With the help of the literature search and further data collection, Stern then related her reactions to those patients feel when they enter the strange and unusual world of the health care field. The concept of culture shock (Stern & Cousins, 1982) proved to be a useful one for further studies.

Connections with Past Study

The variables discovered in a grounded theory study connect with other studies and with the social world outside the study. Once you discover the core variable, you see it everywhere.

Role expectations learned in a particular culture, may be quite different and shocking in another cultural context. In a second look at role expectations in stepfather families, Stern, now sensitized by the Pilipino study, discovered a concept she called "individual family culture" (Stern, 1982b). She explains that, "A family may be called a microcultural unit" (p. 27). Family members have separate and important rules for behaviors and perceptions of roles. Thus, when a woman with a child remarries, all parties involved experience culture shock at what to them are strange and unusual individual family cultural norms of the new family members.

The discovery of the concept of individual family culture became possible after the discovery of cultural variables in the Pilipino study. If we consider the family members to be from different cultures, and relate that to the culture shock Pilipino immigrants experience, we understand that at first family members may be shocked at what they consider improper behavior. In time, some stepfather families develop adaptive behavior like the Pilipino woman in Galveston who realized that, "It's okay to be just as rude as the Americans." Thus, Stern recognized "a known principle in disguise" (Blakeslee, 1980, p. 48).

Meta-Analysis

Webster defines the term meta as, ". . . organized or specialized in form . . . more comprehensive: transcending" (Woolf, 1977, p. 721). The word meta-analysis is taken from a computer methodology described by O'Flynn (1982). Meta-analysis is a comparison of findings from several studies. As O'Flynn explains, it is ". . . the integration of findings, the analysis of analyses . . ." (p. 314). We analyzed the findings from seven grounded theory studies in a meta-analysis called, "Self-Care from the Patient's Perspective: Issues of Culture Shock and Control." Theoretical Analysis (Stern, 1983) and Case Study (Harris, 1983). In this study, the concept of culture shock, between client and nurse, helped to bind the data together. The covariable, showing respect, provided a way of overcoming the shock.

CONCLUSION

In this chapter we presented what we think is a lucid description of the uses of grounded theory in studying cultures. The natural thought processes of the human mind have been introduced and interwoven in attempting to "make sense of it all." To be meaningful and functional, a theory must make sense to thinking human beings, and must spark feelings of identification in everyone.

REFERENCES

Artinian, B. M.(1982). Conceptual mapping: Development of the strategy. *Western Journal of Nursing Research, 4*(4), 379–393.

Blakeslee, T. R. (1980). *The right brain.* Garden City, NY: Anchor/Doubleday.

Brocato, C. (1982). *Right and left brain nursing: Pain assessment on an orthopedic ward.* Unpublished Master's thesis, Northwestern State University of Louisiana, College of Nursing, Shreveport, Louisiana.

Clinton, J. (1982). Ethnicity: The development of an empirical construct for cross-cultural health research. *Western Journal of Nursing Research, 4*(3), 281–300.

Cousins, M. E. B. (1981). *Development of an affiliation scale: Field testing and factor analysis.* Unpublished Master's thesis, Northwestern State University of Louisiana, College of Nursing, Shreveport, Louisiana.

DeMeneses, M. (1980). Split brain theory: Implications for nurse educators. *Nursing Outlook, 28*(7), 441–443.

Denzin, N. K. (1970). *Sociological methodology.* Chicago: Aldine.

Glaser, B. G., & Strauss, A. L. (1967). *The discovery of grounded theory.* Chicago: Aldine.

Glaser, B. G. (1978). *Theoretical sensitivity.* Mill Valley, CA: Sociology Press.

Harris, C. C. (1983, March 19). *Self-care from the patient's perspective: Issues of culture shock and control.* Case Study. Presented to the Society for Applied Anthropology, Annual Meeting, San Diego, California.

Hartmann, F. (1975). Untitled paper. In H. A. Krebs & J. H. Shelly (Eds.) *The creative process in science and medicine.* New York: American Elsevier.

Koestler, A. (1959). *The sleepwalkers.* London: Hutchinson.

Koestler, A. (1964). *The act of creation.* New York: Dell.

Krassen-Maxwell, E. (1979). Modeling life: A qualitative analysis of the dynamic relationship between elderly models and their protegees (Doctoral dissertation, University of California, San Francisco, 1979). *Dissertation Abstracts International,* 1979.

Lewis, J. D. (1979). *Management of chronic hypertension by black clients.* Unpublished doctoral dissertation, University of California, San Francisco.

Louie, T. (1975). *The pragmatic context: A Chinese-American example of defining and managing illness.* Unpublished doctoral dissertation, University of California, San Francisco.

Maxwell, E. K., & Maxwell, R. J. (1980). Search and research in ethnography. *Behavior Science Research, 15*(3), 219–243.

Munhall, P. L. (1982). Nursing philosophy and nursing research: In apposition or opposition? *Nursing Research, 31*(3), 176–177, 181.

O'Brien, M. C. (1982, April). Pragmatic survivorism: Behavior patterns affecting low-level wellness among minority group members. *Advances in Nursing Science,* 26–30.

O'Flynn, A. J. (1982). Meta-analysis. *Nursing Research, 31*(5), 314–316.

Oiler, C. (1982). The phenomenological approach in nursing research. *Nursing Research, 31*(3), 178–181.

Pyles, S. H. (1981). *Assessments related to cardiogenic shock: Discovery of nursing gestalt.* Unpublished Master's thesis, Northwestern State University of Louisiana, College of Nursing, Shreveport.

Pyles, S. H. (1982a). *Discovery of nursing gestalt in critical care nursing: The importance of the Gray Gorilla Syndrome.* Paper presented to the Second Annual Research Conference co-sponsored by the Southern Council on Collegiate Education for Nursing, and University of Alabama at Birmingham, School of Nursing, Birmingham.

Pyles, S. H. (1982b). *Role of critical care nurses in the early detection and prevention of cardiogenic shock: Discovery of the weak link.* Paper presented to the Third Annual Research Conference, co-sponsored by Alpha Delta Chapter, Sigma Theta Tau, and the University of Texas at Galveston, School of Nursing, Galveston.

Pyles, S. H. (1983, March). *Effects of nurse-physician communication in the early detection and prevention of cardiogenic shock.* Paper presented to the Second Annual Research Conference, co-sponsored by Beta Chi Chapter of Sigma Theta Tau and Northwestern State University, College of Nursing, Shreveport, Louisiana.

Pyles, S. H., & Stern, P. N. (1983). Discovery of nursing gestalt in critical care nursing: The importance of the Gray Gorilla Syndrome. *Image: The Journal of Nursing Scholarship, 15*(2), 51–57.

Scott, M. D. S. (1982a). *Childbearing beliefs of northern Louisiana blacks.* Unpublished Master's Thesis. Northwestern State University of Louisiana, College of Nursing, Shreveport, Louisiana.

Scott, M. D. (1982b). Childbearing beliefs of northern Louisiana blacks. Presented to the Eighth Annual Transcultural Nursing Society Conference, Atlanta, GA.

Scott, M. D., & Stern, P. N. (1983). The ethno market theory: Factors influencing childbearing health practices of northern Louisiana black women. In C. N. Uhl & J. Uhl (Eds.) *Proceedings of the Eighth Annual Transcultural Nursing Society Conference.*

Stern, P. N. (1980). Grounded theory methodology: Its uses and processes. *Image, 12*(1), 20–23.

Stern, P. N. (1981). Solving problems of cross-cultural health teaching: The Filipino childbearing family. *Image, 13*(2), 47–50.

Stern, P. N. (1982a). A comparison of culturally-approved behaviors and beliefs between Pilipina-immigrant women, American-born, dominant culture women, and Western female nurses: Religiosity of health care. In P. Morley (Ed.) *Proceedings of the Seventh Annual Transcultural Nursing Society Meeting.* Salt Lake City: University of Utah Press.

Stern, P. N. (1982b). Conflicting family culture: An impediment to integration in stepfather families. *Journal of Psychosocial Nursing and Mental Health Services, 20*(10), 27–33.

Stern, P. N. (1983). Self-care from the patient's perspective: Issues of culture shock and control. Theoretical analysis. Presented to the Society for Applied Anthropology, Annual Meeting, San Diego, CA.

Stern, P. N., Allen, L. M., & Moxley, P. A. (1982). The nurse as grounded theorist: History process and uses. *Review Journal of Philosophy and Social Science, 7*(142), 200–215.

Stern, P. N., & Cousins, M. E. B. (1982). Culture shock as a positive force: Surviving West Coast to northern Louisiana relocation. In C. N. Uhl & J. Uhl (Eds.), *Published Proceedings of the Seventh Annual Transcultural Nursing Conference.* Salt Lake City: University of Utah.

Stern, P. N., Tilden, V. P., & Maxwell, E. K. (1980). Culturally-induced stress during childbearing: The Pilipino-American experience. *Issues in Health Care of Women, 2*(3–4), 67–81.

Swanson, J. M., & Chenitz, W. C. (1982). Why qualitative research in nursing? *Nursing Outlook, 30*(4), 241–245.

Wadd, L. (1983). Vietnamese postpartum practices; implications for nursing in the hospital setting. *JOGN, 12*(4), 252–258.

Wilson, H. S. (1977). Limited intrusion-social control of outsiders in a healing community. *Nursing Research, 26*(2), 103–111.

Woolf, H. B. (Ed.). (1977). *Webster's new collegiate dictionary.* Springfield, MA: Merriam.

BIBLIOGRAPHY

Blumer, H. (1969). *Symbolic interactionism.* Englewood Cliffs, NJ: Prentice-Hall.

Conway, M. E. (1978). Theoretical approaches to the study of roles. In M. E. Hardy & M. E. Conway (Eds.), *Role theory: Perspectives for health professionals,* New York: Appleton Century Crofts.

De Millo, R. A., Lipton, R. J., & Perlis, R. J. (1979). Social processes and proofs of theorems and programs. *Communications of the Association for Computing Machinery, 22*(5), 271–280.

Diers, D. (1979). *Research in nursing practice.* Philadelphia: Lippincott.

Harris, C. C. (1982). Circumcision: A cultural decision. In C. N. Uhl & J. Uhl (Eds.) Proceedings of the Seventh Annual Transcultural Nursing Society Conference, Salt Lake City: University of Utah Press.

Homans, G. C. (1950). *The human group.* New York: Harcourt, Brace & World.

Homans, G. C. (1961). *Social behavior: Its elementary forms.* New York: Harcourt, Brace & World.

Lofland, J. (1971). *Analyzing social settings.* Belmont, CA: Wadsworth.

Ludemann, R. (1979). The paradoxical nature of nursing research. *Image, 11*(1), 2–8.

Mead, G. H. (1964). *George Herbert Mead on social psychology.* (Rev. ed.) Chicago: University of Chicago Press.

Rose, A. M. (1974). A systematic summary of symbolic interaction theory. In J. P. Riehl & C. Roy (Eds.) *Conceptual models for nursing practice,* New York: Appleton-Century-Crofts.

Schatzman, L., & Strauss, A. L. (1973). *Field research: Strategies for a natural sociology.* Englewood Cliffs, NJ: Prentice-Hall.

Wilson, H. S. (1977). Limiting intrusion: Social control of outsiders in a healing community. *Nursing Research, 26*(2), 103–110.

THE CULTURAL DECISION–MAKING MODEL:
FOCUS–CIRCUMCISION

Chandice C. Harris, RN, MSN
Doctoral Student in School of Nursing, Parent-Child Coordinator
in Department of Family Medicine, University of Michigan, Ann Arbor

Circumcision is no longer recommended by the American Academy of Pediatrics. However, in the United States, circumcision still prevails. This paper reports on a qualitative design research study that identifies variables that influence the decision to circumcise the male newborn. A cultural decision-making model is presented that predicts and explains decision-making pathways taken by individuals. The value of this model lies in the opportunity for the nurse to assess as well as intervene based on client knowledge deficits as well as cultural values.

That it is right and proper to be circumcised is an assumption of the dominant American culture. The majority of males born are circumcised before they leave the hospital, even though in 1975 the American Academy of Pediatrics reaffirmed the stance "There is no absolute medical indication for routine circumcision of the newborn . . . circumcision of the male neonate cannot be considered an essential component of adequate total health care" (American Academy of Pediatrics, 1975, p. 610). The Academy's edict along with research that demonstrates the fallacy of the procircumcision argument makes circumcision at best a questionable health practice and at worst, a costly life-threatening ritual. Even more important are the cultural processes that influence the circumcision decision and serve to "disfranchise" males based on the presence of a foreskin.

Circumcision is the most frequently performed surgical procedure in the United States. Currently, in the U.S., 80–99% of newborn males are circumcised (Wirth, 1980), though Wiener (1980, p. 36)

Some of the material presented in this paper originally appeared in the published proceedings of the *Seventh Annual Transcultural Nursing Society Conference,* University of Utah Press, Salt Lake City (1981) under the title "Circumcision: A Cultural Decision."

reports a low of 30% for infants born at home or in alternative birth settings. Still, these rates far surpass other countries where circumcision is viewed as unnecessary, such as in Canada, England, and Sweden (Wirth, 1980). This study addresses the research question, "What variables influence parents' decisions to circumcise or not to circumcise their newborn?"

NEED FOR THE STUDY

The study is seen as important for the following reasons. In 1859, Florence Nightingale promoted the idea that nursing was concerned with discovering and reinforcing nature's "laws of health" (Nightingale, 1859/1970, p. 6). One such "law of health" is that the uncircumcised state is a natural, not pathological condition. There now exists ample scientific evidence to discard the act of circumcision as a health practice. Not so clear are the cultural processes that influence the social need for the circumcision act. Because maternal-child nursing practice requires teaching and counseling the client about their circumcision choice, along with assisting with the procedure, scientific as well as transcultural enlightment of the nurse is necessary (Harris & Stern, 1981).

At present, many health professionals act as "cultural imposers" by denying circumcision to some subcultures who desire the procedure, and promoting circumcision to others who are uncertain as to the need for the procedure (Leininger, 1979, p. 11; Aamodt, 1978). In fact, many doctors and nurses asked me "Why research circumcision? It's such a little thing . . ." (no pun intended). I have observed this "little thing" act as an additional stressor, especially during the postpartum period, when parents are trying to make a decision that they feel will affect their child for a lifetime. Furthermore, Dickoff, James, and Semradek (1975) suggest that "Nursing reality from the consumer's view point is a madhouse world of horrors" (p. 86). They propose that nursing research be evaluated as to "payoff," that is, research in nursing that results in improved patient care processes in the health system (p. 84). It is believed that this study on circumcision will shed light on this controversial cultural and health practice with the final result being an opportunity for improved care for infants and their parents.

BACKGROUND INFORMATION

Around the turn of the century, the status of circumcision changed from a religious rite to a common surgical procedure. In

1891, a physician, Remondino, stated that the foreskin was a "dangerous relic of a far-distant prehistoric age," designed to protect unclothed early man from "bark, brambles, and insect bites."

Historically, the five main reasons for circumcision include: 1) an adolescent initiation rite of passage and test of manhood through torture and pain; 2) a personal sacrifice in a religious ritual; 3) an act to mark, torture, and humiliate slaves and defeated warriors; 4) conforming with hygienic and cosmetic values; and 5) a response to the antimasturbation hysteria of the late 1800s (that is, if the child has to wash under the foreskin, he might learn to masturbate). Even today, many of these reasons are used, but with a slightly different context in language and custom.

Ritual

Woven throughout the history of circumcision is ritual psychoanalytic theory and stigma. Transculturally, rituals are rich in symbolism. The symbolism of circumcision hinges on the absence of a foreskin which implies that more than a simple operation has taken place. Especially in America, it suggests that a well accepted "ritual" has occurred. The term "ritual," according to Gluckman (1975, p. 1) is used to describe many different kinds of phenomena of a repetitive, almost obsessive nature.

When approved by a certain culture, ritual can become standardized, repetitive, and prescribed. That is, cultural rules command that the ritual be performed (Gluckman, 1975, p. 4, 14). Such rules were especially evident in past years when hospitals routinely circumcised newborns, often without informed parental consent.

Most rituals signify a rite of passage and convey a sense of belonging. When a culture accepts a ritual of another culture, it signifies a desire for status passage, or "Keeping up with the Joneses." In the United States, "the Joneses" are the norms, beliefs, and values of the dominant American culture (Glaser & Strauss, 1971). This includes the tradition of circumcision.

Psychoanalytic Theory

Another aspect of circumcision is embodied in the Freudian theory of psychological processes existing between the mother, child, and father. Shrouded in misogyny, these suppositions explain circumcision as a ritual of matriarchal control, a measure to resolve the Oedipal conflict, and a symbolic solution to man's envy of the womb and fear of that envy (Bettelheim, 1954; Gluckman, 1975, p. 6; Kita-hara, 1976; Ostow, 1970).

Stigma

Either society's value of Freud's theory, or the actual existence of said processes has resulted in a foreskin stigma. In subtle and overt ways, the uncircumcised male is stigmatized by the dominant American culture. Fear of stigma leads American parents to elect circumcision. As Cogan (1981, p. 1) points out, there is no American Academy of Pediatrics directive on the management of cultural pressures and potential identity problems generated in the locker room or in the family system due to this stigma.

Clearly, the brunt of the stigma is experienced by the child, not by the parents who made the choice. In the words of one of my chief informants, who is an uncircumcised urban white, "I think there is psychological trauma when you are not circumcised. I went through gym class, being in the locker room. There were no remarks, but I felt different . . ." But not all uncircumcised men in the dominant American culture that were interviewed felt this way. Some related a feeling of superiority, that he possessed something better than being circumcised. Goffman (1963) in his book *Stigma,* explains this attitude as follows:

> It seems possible for an individual to fail to live up to what we effectively demand of him and yet be relatively untouched by this failure; insulated by his alienation, protected by identity beliefs of his own, he feels that he is a full-fledged normal human being, and that we are the ones that are not quite human (p. 6).

Those uncircumcised males or parents of uncircumcised males who do feel stigmatized by the dominant American culture, may attempt to "cover" or restrict the display of the stigma, similar to the idea behind a rhinoplasty or mammoplasty (Goffman, 1963, p. 102). The usual situation is the "circumcision rider" attached to another surgical procedure. Examples of this include the 4-year-old who receives a circumcision along with a tonsillectomy or the 40-year-old who is circumcised along with a vasectomy. What often results is the absence of a fully formal status, that is a circumcised male but one who is according to Goffman (1963), "Someone with a record of having corrected a particular blemish" (p. 102). It is the old horror story, "He had to be circumcised at 40!"

The application of the theory of stigma to noncircumcision may seem tenuous, but I was amazed at how this state was degraded. The expressions "dirty," "bad," "unclean," "tends to masturbate," "preoccupied with sex," and so on surfaced again and again.

Major influences on the development of the foreskin stigma are the myths that make circumcision a necessity. Research exposes these myths, yet the findings are not well distributed nor accepted by the dominant American culture. Concisely, these findings are as follows:

1) Newborns are born with fused foreskins.
2) The foreskin gradually separates. Complete separation may not occur until near puberty.
3) Smegma is most often nonexistent in children.
4) Forced retraction of the foreskin (often done by caretakers) produces scar tissue.
5) Scar tissue produces adhesions.
6) Adhesions make circumcision necessary (a "Catch 22" situation).
7) Cancer of the prostate, cervix, and penis is directly related to personal hygiene, not the presence or lack of a foreskin (Harris & Stern, 1981).

METHODOLOGY

This study was conducted using a naturalistic approach, grounded theory. According to Stern (1980), grounded theory is particularly useful when a new perspective on a familiar situation is needed. Especially in America, the circumcision of newborns is a familiar situation. However a new perspective is now needed because of the American Academy of Pediatrics stance on circumcision.

Background information for this study included several theoretical frameworks relevant to circumcision. Wilson (1977, p. 110) suggests "there are several ways of working with existing theory. . . . Grounded theory offers [an] alternative. . . . that of transcending or bringing parts of other theories into a new, overriding theory." Diers (1979) supports such theory building studies to provide a much needed foundation for health-related causal and experimental research designs.

Data Collection

Data was collected with open, free flowing, and directed interviews. The majority of data represents approximately 60 hours of participant-observation study in north Louisiana. The interviews were conducted at numerous sites and times according to the subject's convenience. At first, the interviews were open and free flowing. As the processes emerged, the interviews became more directed. The interviews were hand recorded verbatim, then later typed for analysis.

Sources of Data

Initially the sources of data were new parents, nursery nurses, and pediatricians. As the processes of the theory emerged, theoretical sampling included pregnant women and couples, parents or older children, urologists, obstetricians, general practitioners, pediatric nurse practitioners, community health nurses, certified nurse midwives, and men and women of various ages. The literature provided an additional source of information.

It is important to emphasize that data from the grounded theory approach is qualitative, not numerative, with hypotheses generated, not tested. Therefore, demographic data, personality factors, and intelligence quotients are not relevant to the study.

Data Analysis

With grounded theory, analyzing the data is a constant, comparative, cognitive process similar to a matrix computer-analyzed design. That is, every individual datum is examined in reference to all other data and to the emerging categories and processes. As themes are discovered, further data collection serves to strengthen and refine these themes. According to Wilson (1977), data are interrelated for "causes, contexts, contingencies, consequences, covariances, conditions, mutual effects, cutting points, degrees, and types" (p. 109). The resultant hypotheses yield a molecular instead of a direct causal relationship. The theorists of grounded theory, Glaser and Strauss (1967, p. 118) refer to this as a "dense" theoretical schema. The credibility of this resultant schema is advanced by the "goodness of fit" the theory has for the real world. It is the "integration, relevance and workability" of the theory that promotes its significance (Glaser, 1978, p. 134).

RESEARCH FINDINGS

In this study, the substantive area is circumcision of newborns under conditions existing in the lay and health culture. The categories named circumcision reasoning, cultural decision-making, and cultural franchising were discovered and are shown in Figure 1.

Circumcision Reasoning

First, the category of circumcision reasoning is presented. The major reasons to circumcise one's child are the same as the reasons to avoid circumcision; for instance the reason "medical advice" was used by both groups. However, the way in which these reasons are defined in the reality of the parent differs markedly from family to family and culture to culture. MacKay (1978, p. 179) explains cultural patterns as designs not only for reality perceptions, but also for constructing that reality. Subjects gave evidence of how they had constructed their reality through their reasons for and against the practice of circumcision. Their answers were categorized into nine main reasons as shown in Figure 2. The emphasis of this report focuses on the reasons to circumcise.

Sign of Manhood
The most common reason to circumcise was "So he will look like his daddy" or "brother." An additional theme of this line of

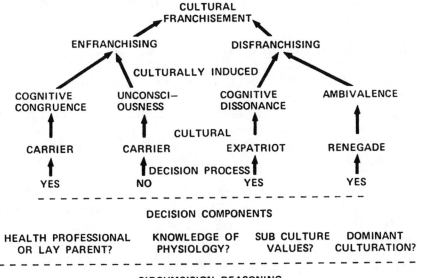

Figure 1. Components of circumcision reasoning.

CIRCUMCISION REASONING	
To Circumcise	**Not To Circumcise**
1. Sign of Manhood	1. Sign of Manhood
2. Culturally Induced Unconsciousness	2. Culturally Induced Unconsciousness
3. No Harm, No Pain	3. Traumatic / Dangerous
4. Sex Worries	4. Sex Worries
5. Hygienic / Cosmetic / Comfort	5. Hygienic / Cosmetic / Comfort
6. Guidance From Bible	6. Guidance From Bible
7. Playing It Safe	7. Playing It Safe
8. Cultural / Sentimental Order	8. Cultural / Sentimental Order
9. Medical Advice	9. Medical Advice

Figure 2. Balance of factors in circumcision reasoning.

reasoning was explained by one father's words, "Even if it hurts, he has to go through it. . . . One day he will thank me." It was interesting to observe the strong emotions evoked, especially in the Anglo male, when told circumcision was no longer recommended. As one informant stated, "It's part of being a man in a man's world. . . . My father was circumcised, I am, and my son will be." This need for the circumcised sign of manhood was reflected in the words of one of my chief informants who said, "Men are put down by those who have [been circumcised]. All males should be, then they have things in common."

Culturally Induced Unconsciousness

The existence of culturally caused or induced unconsciousness was evident in the data (Aamodt, 1978). Such reasoning was . . . "You don't stop to question what has always been done" and "We didn't even talk about it, we just assumed it would be done." Most parents are never in a position to think about, discuss, or question circumcision. There is no need. Due to culturally induced unconsciousness, the child will be circumcised, period.

No Harm, No Pain

As one informant stated, "There are less problems if it is done early. It's bad on a grown man. It can cause him to have problems with sex." Or as another said, "It's better to do it when they're a baby, it doesn't hurt." Also expressed was "There are no nerve endings. Babies don't feel it like a grown man does."

Contrary to these beliefs, research demonstrates that during and following circumcision, newborns show behaviors that when observed in an adult are diagnosed as pain. These include crying, changes in sleep-wake states and feeding patterns, and significant increases in the endocrine response (Anders & Chalemian, 1974; Talbert, 1976). However, since newborns are unable to verbalize this distress, some lay persons as well as health professionals believe that pain is not experienced during the procedure.

Likewise, the issue of harm to newborn is mostly denied. The fact is that 1 out of 500 circumcisions threaten the life of the neonate while few (less than two per million procedures) actually result in death. However, these numbers are being challenged due to the connection between circumcision and neonatal sepsis, a leading cause of neonatal death (McHugh, 1981; Cogan, 1981).

Indeed, males who undergo circumcision later in life do report marked physical and psychological suffering. It is postulated however, that this response occurs because in America, adult circumcision is a mistimed cultural event. Ozturk (1973) reports that in Turkey, children are circumcised between 3–7 years of age without anesthesia. Contrary to the predictable psychological effects of the operation at this age, namely castration anxiety, Ozturk discovered that the societal preparatory experience and meaning overrode such effects. These findings are interesting when applied to the American adult male being circumcised. The dominant American culture ignores, exaggerates, or makes this experience the brunt of jokes. Meanwhile it is interesting that a similar invasive procedure, female episiotomy, has not (until recently) received the notoriety of adult male circumcision. Whether this is due to "woman's long suffering role" or the cultural sanction of episiotomy is not clear.

Sex Worries

Frequently mentioned reasons for advocating circumcision referred to sexual concerns, both for the adult sexuality of the child and his relationship to his mother and father. Mostly, circumcision was viewed as a method to prevent masturbation or promiscuity in sexual matters. One father stated, "It will make it last longer." A mother related, "I had him circumcised when he was two because he started playing with himself." Also I was informed, "Men who are circumcised are able to control themselves; it prevents premature ejaculation." It is interesting that a similar operation, female circumcision is prescribed in America for the opposite effect, namely to cure frigidity (Wollman, 1974). In Egypt, female circumcision is practiced to attenuate the female sexual response (Assaad, 1980).

The theme of sex also worries concerned mothers careing for their sons. As best explained by one female informant, "The child might remember his mother cleaning under the foreskin. Mother has no business doing that." This theme, found across cultures, exposed a fear of an incestuous nature attached to the uncircumcised state.

Hygienic, Comfort, and Cosmetic

The argument procircumcision for reasons of hygiene, comfort, and "beauty" is *greatly* supported by the dominant American culture. First, hygiene can be a problem, especially for individuals who do not practice adequate hygiene due to cultural factors or lack of bathing facilities and supplies. As one 56-year-old male informant explained, "We took a bath a week and you best not be caught washing below the water line. And mom certainly didn't [help with hygienic care]. It wasn't right."

War-associated conditions were also mentioned by some informants, because of the lack of opportunity to cleanse the body during the World War II, Korean, and Vietnam conflicts. However, one urologist interviewed claimed that circumcised males suffer equally in such circumstances, due to irritation of the glans, and of the perineal area in general.

In all, the need for hygiene relates to the occurrence of smegma. Smegma is composed of both a lubricating fluid secreted by the glands of the inner surface of the prepuce (or clitoral hood) and desquamated epithelial cells. This composition has been implicated as carcinogenic, however recent studies have failed to demonstrate this causal relationship. It is important to point out that women also produce smegma. Nurse informants discussed the poor hygiene practices of elderly males. As one said, "A man of 70 is not worried about cleaning himself." Likewise, elderly females suffer some of these same problems, but with more available female care takers, female hygienic care is provided without the "taboo" associated with a female nurse caring for a male.

Comfort reasons were attached to the idea that a "tight" foreskin "bothered" the child. One mother stated that as her son was toilet training, he would "grab at his penis" when he needed to urinate. This she attributed to a "tight skin." Hoever, even after circumcision, the child continued this behavior until full bladder training was achieved.

Finally, the cosmetic appeal of circumcision is best explained by the phrase "Beauty is in the eye of the beholder." In America, the beholder is the dominant culture that has advanced the notion that the circumcised penis is more aesthetic. It is as Leitch (1970) states, "The exposed glans is the fashion" (p. 59). However, in other countries, circumcision is viewed as a barbarous practice that leaves the male disfigured. This is much the same view that an American might have toward female circumcision in some cultures.

As a historical note, the Greeks (A.D. 14–37) in their quest for Christianity balked at the rabbinical directions to undergo circumcision. To meet a consumer need, a "decircumcision" procedure was developed to reconstruct the prepuce after the Greek male was circumcised. This need related to the Greek's love of the natural beauty of the human body (Rubin, 1978).

Guidance from the Bible

Many informants cited the teachings of the Bible as their motivation for circumcision. One informant stated, "My mother regretted not having my four brothers circumcised. She believes from the Bible. . . . Boy babies having to be or they're unclean. She worried about what the Bible said. She prays for my brothers to go to heaven anyway."

Unfortunately, the Bible has been misread and misquoted concerning circumcision. The religious circumcision requirement is associated with Judaism exclusively. Yet, Jewish religious tradition has had the greatest influence on the practice of circumcision in America. The Jewish biblical heritage of the covenant of circumcision addresses the chosen people:

> And God said unto Abraham. . . . This is my covenant, which ye shall keep, between me and you and thy seed after thee; Every man child among you shall be circumcised. . . . And the uncircumcised man child whose flesh of his foreskin is not circumcised, that soul shall be cut off from his people; he hath broken my covenant (Gen. 17:9-14).

One can appreciate the importance of the act to the Jewish people. This covenant was and still is a source of confusion, especially when interpreted to apply to individuals not of the Jewish faith. Such a situation was recorded in the Bible when the Jews suggested the lack of circumcision among the Gentiles excised them from the faith. Apostle Paul's advice in the New Testament cleared up this concern:

> And put no difference between us [the Jews] and them [the Gentiles], purifying their hearts by faith (Acts, 15:9). . . . Is any man called [to the faith] being circumcised: Let him not become uncircumcised. I any called in [to the faith] uncircumcised: Let him not be circumcised (1 Corinthians, 7:18).

These passages implied that God wanted evidence of faith, not merely circumcision, from the Gentiles, the concept of "circumcision of the heart." It is interesting then, that one of the main reasons given by parents today who are not Jewish is, "It says to do it in the Bible . . . doesn't it?"

Playing It Safe

Some parents elect to have their sons circumcised even when they are uncertain as to the need. This need to "play it safe" was evident in the data from one mother who stated, "I know that it's not needed, but I worried. I decided to have it done just in case something went wrong." There are many other examples of "playing it safe" such as infant baptism by agnostic parents and the educated woman not raising her hands above her head during pregnancy. Playing it safe allows the individual to "ward off" danger, or in a way, bargain with fate. That is, "If I have my son circumcised, he won't have problems." This reasoning is closely associated with the next reason, that of sentimental order.

Cultural Sentimental Order

Sentimental order is an emotional attachment to familiar ways of doing things (Stern, 1982). The emotion of sentimental order compels one to ascription. As an example, one couple interviewed was on the waiting list to adopt a boy baby. In our area, the relinquished infant is circumcised before his adoptive parents are notified. Since this adoptive father was uncircumcised and adamantly against circumcision, the couple changed their preference to a girl baby.

Health professionals also "suffer" from the effects of sentimental order. One pediatrician, whose spouse was pregnant, said, "I don't know what I'll do if it's a boy. It just seems right to circumcise my son, even though I know it's not necessary to do it." Some of the health professionals, in order to save professional "face," placed responsibility on the spouse for electing circumcision for their son. In fact, all pediatricians interviewed stated they were against circumcision; however, their children *were* circumcised.

In all, it was discovered that meeting one's sentimental order for circumcision provided comfort to parents and their friends and relatives. Failure to experience this sentimental order led to associated feelings, such as uneasiness, guilt, regret, grief, and a sense of courting disaster.

Medical Advice

While no longer advocated by the Academy, circumcision is still very much valued by some physicians and nurses. One nurse interviewed stated, "I encourage all my friends to have it done when they have a boy. It solves a lot of problems." Some general practitioners, OB–GYNs, and urologists interviewed supported circumcision or forced retraction. As one general practitioner stated, "You have to free the foreskin then teach the mother to keep it back. But some women just won't do it. So the baby has to be circumcised later." However, forced retraction *is not* a therapeutic intervention. The two opposing epithelial surfaces tend to seal together following forced retraction and adhesions form (Harris & Stern, 1981).

Many physicians interviewed mentioned parent and staff pressure to have the circumcision performed. As one said, "The nurse is my worst enemy on this. I get the parents agreeing not to have it done and before I can get back to my office the nurse has talked them into wanting it again. So it's just easier to go ahead and do it." On the other hand, one nurse-mother of boys informed me of intense pressure from her obstetrician to have the circumcision done. "I really had to stand my ground on this" she reported. Health ethno-centrism, which is the health professional's belief that their factual and value systems are always correct, governs medical advice (Mac-kay, 1978). In the case of circumcision, many professionals do not accept the findings that eliminate the need for the procedure. As a urologist stated, "I've never seen a circumcised man with penile cancer. They can't tell me it (circumcision) doesn't prevent cancer."

In all, the reasons to circumcise are varied and have different meanings for each individual parent. Likewise, none of the reasons are based in facts. Value systems and cultural beliefs form the framework of the reasons as described.

Cultural Decision-Making Process

The second category is the cultural decision-making process. As stated by Cogan (1981, p. 1), "Whatever its origin and meaning, circumcision represents a difficult area of decision-making for many prospective parents today, except where unambiguous cultural tradition facilitates decision-making." Most parents experience a decision-making process that hinges on four main states of nature: 1) is the parent a health professional?, 2) does the parent understand the physiology of the foreskin?, 3) does the parent's sub-culture value circumcision?, and 4) does the parent value and ascribe to dominant American cultural prescriptions such as circumcision? This process is depicted in a Cultural Decision-Making Model in Figure 3.

To use the model, the health professional first determines if the parent is a lay person or is affiliated with a health profession. Second, knowledge about physiology of the prepuce and myths is

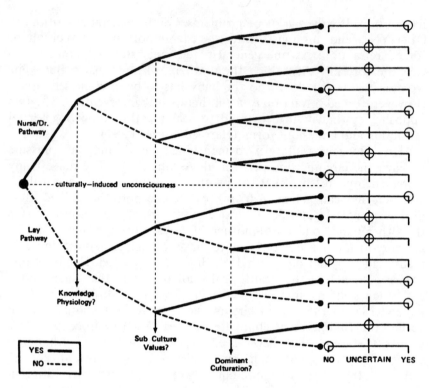

Figure 3. Cultural decision-making model.

assessed. This knowledge causes hesitation in the decision. When given such information, many parents were surprised and it did make the decision more difficult. However, knowing does not assure valuing of such information. As Aamodt (1978) states, "Common sense ways of acting on health and healing situations may appear either to be related or unrelated to a cultural belief system" (p. 10).

Third, in the use of the model, the subcultural beliefs about circumcision are determined. Some groups, such as the American Indians and Hispanics have not traditionally practiced circumcision. Therefore, it is not part of their sentimental order. Similar to an ethnic subculture is what Stern (1982) describes as "individual family culture." This refers to the nuclear and extended family's unique sentimental orders and cultural heritage. While a parent *may* be part of the dominant American culture, there are special influences from the individual family culture.

Finally, the parent's relationship to the dominant American culture is assayed. Valuing the dominant American culture's prescriptions in general implies cultural change or acculturation of the sub-culture parent.

By tracing the pathway in response to the states of nature questions, one arrives at a decision to circumcise, a decision not to circumcise, or uncertainty over the decision. The model predicts the decision-making pathways that individuals take in response to the described states of nature. The value of this model lies in the opportunity for the health professional to assess as well as intervene based on client knowledge deficits and cultural values. Also the model can be used to interrelate across the domains of ethnocentric health practices as an explanatory teaching tool for nurses, physicians, social workers, health educators, and anthropologists.

Cultural Franchise

As the research process advanced, the third category of cultural franchising (see Figure 4) became evident. Parents who elected to have their sons circumcised were accepted or "franchised" by the dominant American cultural network of family, friends, associates, and even health professionals. Those resisting or not following the cultural network were pressured, criticised or "disfranchised." Some sought later circumcision for their child to relieve these pressures.

The outcomes of the decision to circumcise or not to circumcise led to a classification of three main archetypical cultural actors:

1. The cultural carrier—one who follows and promotes cultural norms (Aamodt, 1978); for example, the urban white.
2. The cultural expatriot(ate)—one who is denied access to practicing cultural norms, such as the indigent southern Black.
3. The cultural renegade—one who purposively does not practice cultural norms, for example, the Hispanic or naturalist parent.

These actors' decisions invoked feelings of either cognitive congruence, dissonance, or ambivalence. Congruence is simply agreement between cultural norms and actions. Dissonance implies nonagreement between cultural norms and actions, along with the associated feelings, such as uneasiness, guilt, regret, and a sense of courting disaster. Finally, ambivalence is the alternating emotion of being drawn to, yet at the same time, repelled by cultural norms and actions.

In response to their circumcision choice, the parent and child are enfranchised or disfranchised by their subculture as well as the dominant American culture. The franchise is cultural credibility. It may be described as a cultural credit card—the "American Express" in the

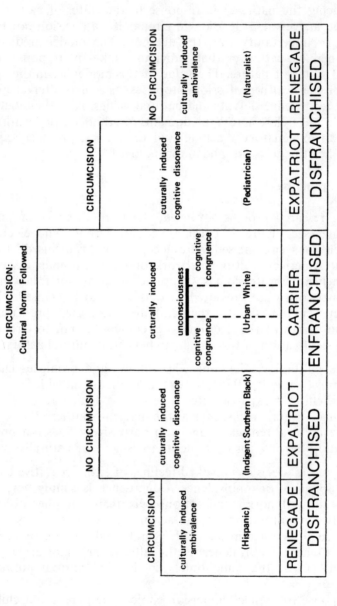

Figure 4. Critical junctures of franchisement.

40

locker room. The best example of this disfranchised process was given by one of my chief informants. This circumcised Anglo father who elected not to have his son circumcised stated:

> When we brought the baby home, my neighbor came over and noticed during a diaper change that my son was not circumcised. He asked me about it. When I told him that we had decided not to have him circumcised, he gave me all of the reasons that we should. He said only poor blacks and farm boys aren't. Once he saw that his pleading was doing no good, he got angry and left.

Specifically, the two main processes of the Cultural Franchise theory are as follows: (a) enfranchising, or the process of extending cultural credibility in response to acceptable behaviors and attitudes, and (b) disfranchising, the process of denying this cultural credibility when cultural norms are not observed.

CONCLUSIONS

In conclusion, I call for a transcultural health setting defined by Aamodt (1978), "as one in which health professionals and clients informed by different cultural, health, and healing systems communicate and resolve their differences in order to meet the needs of the client" (p. 9). As demonstrated in this study, those needs vary in regard to circumcision. The major categories discovered were the reasons for and against electing circumcision, a cultural decision-making process, and the outcomes of the decision to circumcise or not to circumcise, or the Cultural Franchise.

Two clear stances guide client care. One is as Zimmer (1977) states: "When a physician disagrees with the parents on performing the operation but goes along with their decision, this is not medical leadership" (p. 505). This viewpoint directs health professionals to inform parents and encourage them strongly not to have their child circumcised or even not to offer the procedure.

The second viewpoint allows a less rigid alignment with scientific knowledge. That is, circumcision is an acceptable practice based on cultural values. As Leininger (1979) suggests:

> Ritualized ethno-caring activities can have highly therapeutic benefits to clients and their families and should not be readily modified or disbanded as "too routine" and "nontherapeutic" caring measures (p. 24).

Therefore, since circumcision is a relatively safe practice, culture might be the deciding factor. The teaching, anticipatory guidance, and actual procedure must be in tune with "cultural boundedness," namely the "relationship between a cultural system and a cultural carrier" (Aamodt, 1978, p. 8). In this way, the health professional is a caring and perceptive cultural broker. The assessment needed to provide this harmony can be completed using the described Cultural Decision-Making Model.

The theory of the Cultural Franchise is grounded in the experiences of parents, health professionals, and the child. Finally, a major discovery of this study was that the truly disfranchised individual is the circumcised son of the enfranchised parent. He has no options and no freedom to change his state.

REFERENCES

Aamodt, A. (1978). Culture. In A. Clark (Ed.), *Cultural-childbearing-health professionals*. Philadelphia: Davis.

American Academy of Pediatrics. (1975). Report of the ad hoc task force on circumcision. *Pediatrics, 56,* 610–611.

Anders, T., & Chalemian, R. (1974). The effects of circumcision on sleep-wake states in human neonates. *Psychosomatic Medicine, 36,* 174–179.

Assaad, M. (1980). Female circumcision in Egypt: Social implications, current research, and prospects for change. *Studies in Family Planning, 11*(1), 3–16.

Bettelheim, B. (1954). *Symbolic wounds: Puberty rites and the envious male.* New York: Free Press.

Cogan, R. (1981). Circumcision. *ICEA Review, 5*(1), 1–7.

Dickoff, J., James, P., & Semradek, J. (1975). 8-4 Research part I: A stance for nursing research—Tenacity or inquiry. *Nursing Research, 24*(2), 84–88.

Diers, D. (1979). *Research in nursing practice.* Philadelphia: Lippincott.

Glaser, B. (1978). *Theoretical sensitivity.* Mill Valley, CA: Sociology Press.

Glaser, B., & Strauss, A. (1967). *The discovery of grounded theory: Strategies for qualitive research.* Chicago: Aldine.

Glaser, B., & Strauss, A. (1971). *Status passage.* Chicago: Aldine.

Gluckman, M. (1975). Specificity of social—Anthropological studies of ritual. *Mental Health Society, 2,* 1–17.

Goffman, E. (1963). *Stigma: Notes on the management of spoiled identity.* Englewood Cliffs, NJ: Prentice-Hall.

Harris, C., & Stern, P. (1981). Care of the prepuce in the uncircumcised child: Reinforcing nature's laws of health. *Issues in Comprehensive Pediatric Nursing, 5*(4), 233–242.

Kitahara, M. (1975). A cross-cultural test of the Freudian theory of circumcision. *International Journal of Psychoanalytic Psychotherapy, 5,* 535–546.

Leininger, M. (1979). *Transcultural nursing.* New York: Masson.

Leitch, I. (1970). Circumcision: A continuing enigma. *Austrian Pediatrics, 6,* 59.

MacKay, S. (1978). Cultural factors as a source of influence on the health professions. In M. Hardy & M. Conway (Eds.), *Role theory—Perspectives for health professionals.* New York: Appleton-Century-Crofts.

McHugh, M. (1981). Circumcision–Is it ever necessary? *Irish Medical Journal, 74*(2), 55–56.

Nightingale, F. (1859/1970). *Notes on nursing: What it is, and what it is not.* (2nd ed.), London: Duckworth.

Ostow, M. (1970). Parent's hostility to their children. *Israel Annals of Psychiatry and Related Disciplines, 8*(1), 3–21.

Ozturk, O. (1973). Ritual circumcision and castration anxiety. *Psychiatry, 36,* 49–59.

Remondino, P. (1891/1974). *History of circumcision from the earliest time to the present.* Philadelphia: Davis & AMS.

Rubin, J. (1978). Celsus' decircumcision operation: Medical and historical implications. *Urology, 16*(1), 121–124.

Stern, P. (1980). Grounded theory methodology: Its uses and processes. *Image, 12*(1), 20–23.

Stern, P. (1982). Conflicting family culture: An impediment to integration in stepfather families. *Journal of Psychosocial Nursing, 20*(10), 27–33.

Talbert, L. (1976). Adrenal cortical response to circumcision in the neonate. *Obstetrics Gynecology, 48,* 208–210.

Weiner, R. (1980). Circumcision. *Mothering, 16,* 35–40.

Wilson, H. (1977). Limiting intrusion–Social control of outsiders in a healing community–An illustration of qualitative comparative analysis. *Nursing Research, 26*(2), 103–111.

Wirth, J. (1980). Current circumcision practices: Canada. *Pediatrics, 66*(5), 705–708.

Wollman, L. (1974). Female circumcision. *Journal American Society Psychosomatic Medicine, 20*(4), 130–131.

Zimmer, P. (1977). Modern ritualistic surgery. *Clinical Pediatrics, 16*(6), 503–506.

THE ETHNO-MARKET THEORY: FACTORS INFLUENCING CHILDBEARING HEALTH PRACTICES OF NORTHERN LOUISIANA BLACK WOMEN

Mary Dell Shelton Scott, MS, RN
Southern Arkansas University, Magnolia, Arkansas

Phyllis Noerager Stern, DNS, RN, FAAN
Dalhousie University, Halifax, Nova Scotia

Black women in northern Louisiana either follow the folk beliefs taught to them by elder, follow the prescriptions of the dominant health culture, or balance the advice of these two groups. We discovered that their decisions about which health system they will use are influenced by three factors: the *respect-fear* process that includes the respect shown them by the professional as opposed to the fear they have of breaking traditional taboos; *testing* consisting of trying out new health prescriptions; and *cultural interaction,* that is, the amount and kind of interaction they have had with the dominant culture.

Jane Jones (not her real name), a 20-year-old black woman, just delivered an apparently normal healthy child. It will be 4–6 weeks before Jane will take a tub bath. Even though her hair is nappy and beginning to smell, she will need to wait several weeks before washing it. Jane's aunt would love to hold the baby, but she is menstruating and the family believes that a menstruating woman can give a baby "the stretches."

Would these beliefs, which are considered normal to many southern blacks be thought of as strange by a white nurse? Our experience working in the dominant culture health system leads us to believe that they would.

When this chapter was written Dr. Stern was Professor and Coordinator of Graduate Studies in Maternal-Child & Family Nursing, Northwestern State University College of Nursing, Shreveport, Louisiana. The concepts in this paper were presented in a somewhat different form at the Eighth Annual Transcultural Nursing Society Conference, Atlanta, Georgia, September 1, 1982.

The health care given most of us in the United States, regardless of our personal cultural beliefs, reflects beliefs peculiar to the dominant health care system. Even black nurses working with black clients, offer little help, because they have been taught a new set of norms in schools and institutions, and therefore usually accept only mainstream "scientific" beliefs as valuable.

A knowledge of the cultural practices and beliefs of blacks as they relate to care of the adult woman, childbearing, and childrearing, may assist nurses in accepting and understanding these clients. In this way, black mothers may be able to achieve a more satisfying pregnancy and childrearing outcome. This research addresses the following problems: (a) What are the values and meanings of certain childbearing and childrearing beliefs for a selected number of northern Louisiana black women? (b) How can nurses provide culturally sensitive care for clients who hold these beliefs?

BACKGROUND

Concepts relevant to this study include a historical perspective, the extended black family in relation to the folk medical system, and cross-cultural communication and health teaching.

Blacks were brought to America from West Africa during the 18th century. During the slave years, black women were highly acclaimed for their breeding capability. Most sources agree that blacks were forced to suffer many cruelties (Elkins, 1979; Rodgers-Rose, 1980). One of the stronger black cultural patterns is that of the extended family help system (Greathouse & Miller, 1981). The social network consists of relatives, friends, and neighbors. Staples (1973) stated that the survival of black people is largely due not only to their willingness to help their relatives, but also their concern for their fellow man.

The evolution of a historically grounded extended black family has had significant effects on health beliefs, particularly those relating to childbearing. Often the grandmother is an important figure in the passing of beliefs. Frazier's (1939) classic description of the black grandmother still stands. Frazier contended that it is the black grandmother who guards the generations.

The present study was a direct outgrowth of an investigation of cross-cultural health teaching between Filipino-Americans and Western nurses (Stern, 1981). Findings from that study indicated that styles of approach, custom, and language barriers inhibited cross-cultural health teaching. The Filipino study also indicated that the nurse who showed respect to Filipino clients and valued their health beliefs, enjoyed greater success in transcending cultural barriers. A study of northern Louisiana black childbearing women would yield results that could be compared to the Filipino study and could explore cultural barriers further.

METHOD

We used a Grounded Theory (Glaser & Strauss, 1967) research design to collect and analyze data. The first author, who is black, collected the bulk of the data during 20 in-depth interviews with black women of northern Louisiana who were pregnant at the time of the interview, or who had been pregnant at least once. The age of the women ranged from 14–90 years, and educational level ranged from "some schoolin" through graduate school.

The second author who is non-black participated in the analysis of the data and the writing of the research report. Then both authors checked out the findings for validity with black colleagues and associates.

In the grounded theory approach to research, data are constantly compared with other data as they are collected (Stern, 1980). Processes discovered in the raw data are coded using a system of open codes. Then coded data are compared and grouped into naturally related categories. For example, as we compared data from the interviews, we discovered that women learned folk beliefs from their mothers or other older women; therefore, a category of folk belief repository, in the person of an older woman, was formed. Later, categories were compared and combined until we discovered a substantive theory that explained the situation under study: *The Ethno-Market Theory.*

FINDINGS

Our findings cluster around two major points: (a) Many northern Louisiana blacks have some beliefs that are different from those of the dominant culture health care system; (b) such factors as proximity to other cultures, age, and most importantly, their experience with the dominant culture system, influence the black woman's health care practices regarding herself and her children during early adulthood, pregnancy, and childrearing.

In the first part of this paper, we describe some common beliefs held by northern Louisiana black women. In part two, we describe what we have named the *Ethno-Market Theory.* The Ethno-Market Theory explains how these beliefs are stored, how they are passed on, what processes influence black women to either accept traditional black beliefs, of the dominant culture health system, and identifies the women according to which belief system they accept or "buy."

BELIEFS ABOUT WOMEN AND THEIR CHILDREN

Black women in this study talked with the interviewer about a number of folk beliefs. We chose to present here only those health beliefs that every woman in the study mentioned. What follows then, can be considered a consensual list rather than a comprehensive description of folk health beliefs held by northern Louisiana black women. The following discussion concerns beliefs and their symbolic meanings concerning mestruation, bathing constraints during menstruation and postpartum, pregnancy, diet during pregnancy and postpartum, and care of the infant, including care of the navel, care of thrush, and care of the teething infant. Here and there, for the sake of clarity, we include the so-called scientific health beliefs from the dominant culture. Our general reference for these beliefs is a commonly used nursing text, *Maternity Nursing,* by Reeder, Mastrionni, and Martin (1980). Other sources are cited throughout.

Meaning of Menstruation, Blood Flow, and Lochia

Throughout the study, a special significance was placed on the menstrual flow by our informants. Women called the menarche a "special time," and said, "It meant that I could get pregnant." Terms for menstruation used by the women in the present study are those commonly used by Americans generally; for example, "period," "cycle," "menses," "the curse," and "that time of the month."

Bathing Constraints

Through information gathered from the majority of the subjects, it is clear that the cultural message about bathing and washing one's hair during menstruation or while the flow of lochia persists is to avoid both these activities because bathing and shampooing during these times causes nonspecific but certain illness during old age. Older women, for example, credited their avoidance of bathing and shampooing during menstruation with good health in their later years. All women in the study had been told not to take baths during these times because "their pores were open." Snow (1974) writing about black beliefs explained this hydrophobia by calling it a "preventive" practice. Young girls are strongly advised, according to

Snow, not to wash their hair, take tub baths, go swimming, or sub-
merge their feet in water. At the same time, however, cleanliness is
stressed.

We noted with interest that bathing prohibitions extended beyond
the black population. In an informal survey of our caucasian colleagues, each person could remember a mother, an aunt, or other
older relative who cautioned against bathing and shampooing during
menstruation. Withers (1966), in a survey of southern whites, found
that bathing during the menses may be blamed for insanity or
tuberculosis.

Similar bathing and shampooing constraints pertain while the flow
of lochia persists following childbirth. Women in this study were told
by their mothers or another older woman to avoid taking a bath after
the delivery of the baby for 6 weeks or a month. An informant explained, "It takes a while for the womb to close after the baby comes
so you should not sit in a tub. But you can take a shower." Caution
extended to shampooing. "It used to be 6 weeks before you could
wash your hair" we were told, "now it's just a month that they
[older women] tell you to wait."

Many cultures around the world warn against bathing for a period
following childbirth. In a former study involving Filipinos (Stern,
1981), we found similar bathing prohibitions. In certain Chinese
cultures, it is believed that bathing too soon following childbirth
causes a condition known as postpartum arthritis (Tan, personal
communication, November 10, 1980).

Symbolic Meaning of Menstruation and Its Projected
Effects on Infants

A menstruating woman holds special dangers for a newborn baby.
Every woman told the interviewer that an older family member
warned them that a menstruating woman could give the baby "the
stretches." According to our informants, stretches refers to a condition which affects the baby causing it to pull and strain frequently.
These movements are not related to any apparent physical stimuli.
When asked to describe the baby with the stretches, our informants
told us that the baby seemed "irritable," "fretful," "fussy," " a baby
that cries a lot," and "a baby that stretches a lot."

Any newborn held by a menstruating woman is considered at risk
for developing stretches "until they're 6 weeks old." One 90-year-old
woman explained:

> I never let anybody hold my babies unless I ask them if it's that time of
> the month. If they're having it, then they don't hold my babies because
> I've seen plenty of babies with the stretches.

Nurses were not exempt from giving babies the stretches. A 15-year-old related this incident:

> My sister's baby had to stay in the hospital for a while after he was born because he had the yellow jaundice, and when he got out, he had the stretches. My mother told her one of the nurses in the hospital had been on her period, and had given the baby the stretches.

Beliefs about the effects of menstruation on infants are discussed by Webb (1971). Webb found that black women in the South believe that a newborn child should not be handled by a menstruating woman lest the infant be caused to "strain" (p. 291).

The treatment for stretches is to "take a string off the undergarment of the woman who gave the baby the stretches and tie it around the baby's wrist or ankle." However, if no one knows who gave the baby the stretches, "it just has to wear off."

Care of the Infant

Every society provides special care to protect infants. Black women of northern Louisiana talked about cord care, teething, and thrush.

Care of the Cord

Black women in this study all received instructions on cord care from some health professional, usually a nurse. Nurses suggested that a cord dressing is unnecessary since exposure to air enhances drying of the cord. Generally, nurses told the women to wipe the base of the cord with alcohol daily because alcohol makes the cord dry even more quickly.

Respondents who were in the 20- to 30-year age group usually followed the directions of their nurse. For example, one 28-year-old woman said, "The nurse told me to just clean the navel with alcohol, so I did." Older subjects however—those over 40—and adolescents who lived with their mothers used "bellybands," a white cloth, a "bow" (silver) dollar, and the like, in order to prevent "hernia." This comment was typical:

> My grandmother told me to put a bellyband with a bow dollar on it. This will keep the navel from sticking out, and the baby's back straight.

Concern about umbilical hernia crossed age lines. All women tended to use a bellyband "if the baby's navel stuck out." Sometimes, we were told, "putting the band on the navel and keeping them from crying will make the navel go down."

Treatment for Thrush Mouth

Thrush mouth or candida albicans is a common condition that newborns develop after contact with the causative organism while passing through the birth canal. Babies who develop thrush while in the nursery are usually treated (as of this writing) with some sort of antibiotic drops. Untreated, thrush tends to be self-limiting. Therefore any treatment one tries seems to work. Thus, the treatment black women in our study used, seemed to cure the condition. When asked if anyone had told them that thrush could be self-limiting, women replied that they had not been told this.

Black women in this study told us that the treatment for thrush was for a boy who has never seen his father to blow into the mouth of the infant with thrush. (Thrush was frequently called "thrush" by the respondents even though the interviewer used the word thrush.)

> My auntie's baby had the thrash and she had this man to blow in the baby's mouth and it cured it.... Sure it works. My brother could take a baby from the mother, and when he brought it back, it wouldn't be long before the thrash was gone.

Women set no time limit between treatment and cure. When asked, they said, "Oh, it takes a while," and "You never can tell how long it will take."

Teething

Infants with temporary teeth erupting generally become irritable, have difficulty sleeping, and often refuse to eat. The remedy used to ease the teething infant varied with the age of the woman we talked with. Women past 40 or teens living with their mothers used a dime or penny on a string that hung around the baby's neck. Women in the 20- to 40-year-age group, however, laughed at the idea of money around the baby's neck. "We're not rich enough to have money lying around. We can't even keep money in his piggybank" one woman told us.

The use of a dime or a penny seems to be a variation on the common dominant culture practice of offering a teething baby a chilled metal spoon or a frozen teething ring to ease the irritation of teething. The dimes and pennies around the baby's neck seem to represent an old substitute for a teething ring.

Diet

A good diet cannot guarantee a good pregnancy outcome, but makes an important contribution to it. The nutritional state that a woman brings into pregnancy has a direct bearing on her well-being and on that of her child. The following sections describe some black ethnic regulations for the pregnant or nursing mother. Women most commonly mentioned greens, salt, greasy food, and junk food.

No Greens, No Salt

We found that many northern Louisiana black women restrict from their diets foods that are high in nutritional values and that nurses often advised for a healthy pregnant diet. However, as Powers (1982) maintains, advice that does not accommodate to the life-style, dietary patterns, and beliefs of clients is not likely to be followed. Some of the women in our study avoided foods because of beliefs passed down from generation to generation. "My grand-mother told me not to eat greens until the baby is 6 weeks old" we were told. Another woman told us, "You're not supposed to eat mustard greens after the baby comes because they will kill you. . . . If you're breastfeeding, it will give the baby the colic." Greens are grown in many southern gardens, and therefore are an inexpensive food source of vitamin A, vitamin C, calcium, and iron.

Bohannan (1981) explains that myths have always provided for our most vexing problems and our most treasured solutions. How-ever, when conditions change, perhaps the time-honored principles of the myth are no longer helpful—even harmful. Perhaps the alleged dangers of greens represent just such an outdated myth.

Salt, Greasy Food, Junk Food

Women told us that "greasy foods," "salt," and "junk food" were on their culturally restricted list. For example, "My sister told me that you're not supposed to eat a lot of salt and greasy foods while you're pregnant." Adolescents in the study said their mothers told them to stay away from junk food. One 15-year-old was advised, "My mother told me to eat three balanced meals and drink milk and water and not eat too much sugar."

THE ETHNO–MARKET THEORY

The Ethno-Market Theory, discovered in this study, explains how lay consumers (in this case northern Louisiana black women) ap-proach, and then select their own belief system from the bicultural influences of folk health beliefs, and dominant culture health care "scientific" beliefs. Folk beliefs are passed down through genera-tions. Thus, the older person, mother, or grandmother becomes the repository of folk beliefs. We have named this woman the *cultural warehouse,* because she stores folk remedies for succeeding generations. This woman also becomes the *cultural conveyor* because she teaches these remedies to younger persons, usually younger women. When a client comes in contact with the dominant culture health care system, that client's decision about whether to buy scientific remedies, or the more familiar folk treatments depends to a large measure on certain processes that influence her or his selection. We call these processes, *fear-respect, testing,* and *cultural interaction.* Depending on the outcome of these processes, the client becomes either what we call a *corporate buyer,* a *careful shopper,* or a *cultural buyer.* The dominant health system market place is the hospital, office, health unit, and occasionally during field visits, the client's home. Conversely, the folk market place is the home of the client or the homes of their extended kin. Figure 1 shows a graphic representation of the Ethno-Market Theory.

CULTURAL WAREHOUSE, CULTURAL CONVEYOR

It was discovered in this study that older black women are held responsible for the storing and conveying of folk health treatments. Very early in the study it became clear that either a mother or a mother surrogate passes on folk information to young women about how to care for themselves and their children. One woman explained, "My mother told me what to expect when I got pregnant." Her experience agreed with that of the other women with whom we talked. Ladner (1971) found that many young black girls first discuss

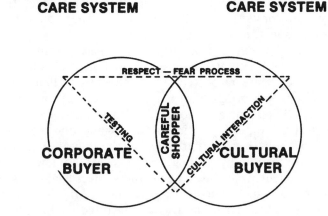

Figure 1. *The Ethno-Market Theory:* Its concepts and processes.

menstruation, kissing, and sexual intercourse with their girlfriends before these topics are discussed with their mothers or other adult females. Data from the present study showed that once young women became pregnant, even if they live away from home, they continue to depend largely on their mother or mother surrogate for advice.

DETERMINING PROCESSES; BUYING INTO THE SYSTEM

Throughout this study, we attempted to find out which processes determine whether the woman follows the traditional beliefs of her family culture or the teachings of the dominant health culture system. We found the dominant processes that influenced her decision to be *respect-fear, testing,* and *cultural interaction.*

Respect-Fear Process

This process is made up of a respect-disrespect continuum, and the development of fear. Respect-disrespect involves the way one is treated in care-seeking situations.

Respect-Disrespect

Showing respect means indicating honor or high esteem for someone. In northern Louisiana, people generally show respect to one another by using the formal address, that is, using last names with the title of Mr., Mrs., or Miss. Older persons are addressed as "sir" or "ma'am." Black women we talked with said that when they entered the dominant culture health arena, they were often addressed by their first names even when they were older than the nurse, physician, or clerk who addressed them. They found this form of address disrespectful.

Showing respect extends to following one's parent's teaching. Since the most influential advice giver in the black family is the mother, her words are respected. When the black client enters the scientific system, she brings with her a great respect for her family's health advice. When nurses or other health professionals belittle or ignore such client values, conflicts result. When one woman asked her physician about her mother's advice, the doctor short-circuited any further discussion by calling these beliefs "old wives' tales." Although the client never brought up the subject again, her respect for her mother was such that she followed her mother's prescriptions not that of the physician. She also felt insulted by the physician's labeling of her mother's advice.

Data from this study indicate that nurses often failed to show their client the respect of an explanation. A woman talked about her delivery experience:

> The doctor hadn't made it there yet and the nurse told me to pant like a puppy dog. She didn't say *why,* so I didn't do it.

When the interviewer explained that the nurse had most likely been trying to avoid a precipitous delivery, the woman said that she would have panted had she known the reason why. "I just didn't want to look stupid," she said.

Women in this study who were not shown respect by the dominant system were not willing to share their beliefs nor take on the system's prescriptions. Consequently, nurses and other providers could not discuss with them the possible benefit or harm of these practices.

Fearing

Many women feared the consequences to themselves and their babies if they failed to follow traditional prescriptions. "I thought my baby would get the stretches if I let a woman on her period hold him" we were told. Other women seemed to fear the dominant health care system. Blacks in this study were very distrustful and suspicious of being used as guinea pigs or being used to perpetuate myths and stereotypes. Their fears are supported in the literature. For example, one of the most inhumane experiments in U.S. history was the Tuskegee study conducted by the United States Public Health Service over a 40-year period. Four hundred black patients infected with syphillis were denied proper treatment in order that scientists could observe the natural effects of the disease. Over 100 black people died as a result of this federally funded health research project (Williams, 1975).

In the present study, fear of experimentation was evident in this comment:

> My friends told me to get the baby out of the hospital because they will experiment with our babies. So I took the baby home.

Other women feared the consequences of not following the dominant health culture. A typical response we heard was, "I was scared my baby would be sick if I didn't do what the nurses said."

Testing

It became apparent that from time to time most of the women in this study had tested some of the traditional and dominant culture beliefs. If they had positive results, they were more apt to challenge another folk belief than if they had negative results. One black nurse explained this testing:

> My mother had told me not to wash my hair while my cycle was on but I did. And the first time I did, I got so sick, I thought I was going to die. It was a while before I tried it again.

Another respondent said, "I was not around my aunt when the baby came so I washed my hair in one week."

One subject had tested the belief but not on herself. She had worked for a white woman who had a new baby and wanted some greens cooked. The respondent said:

> I started to tell her that she shouldn't eat the greens, but I knew that she would laugh at me. So I cooked them and let her eat them. I was scared that she was going to die, but she didn't. So after that I started eating greens after I had my babies.

This "testing" is similar to processes identified by Harrison and Harrison (1971) that included testing, suspicion, and avoidance. These occur in numerous ways: (a) Going to a clinic or health facility, sitting or standing, and simply observing for a period of time without registering, then abruptly leaving; and (b) Sending an older child to the clinic for a one-time treatment. Both of these examples are methods to measure the friendliness and concern of the staff. If the results are unfavorable, family and friends are warned against the clinic.

Cultural Interaction

Whether a woman follows her traditional beliefs or buys part of the standard health care package depends on the quantity and quality of her interaction with other cultures, particularly the dominant white culture. The typical areas that contribute to a woman's relationship to the health care system are education, media exposure, and availability of resources.

Education

Health care materials for the general public are usually written for a sixth-grade reading level. Out of the 20 women interviewed, 70% had a high school education; therefore, they had no difficulty reading pamphlets or books pertaining to pregnancy and infant care. Respondents said that they read pamphlets at the doctor's office and the clinic. For instance, one 25-year-old woman said, "My mother told me some things, but I read pamphlets and books too." One black nurse said, "If I had not gone to nursing school, I would not have questioned some of the things my mother told me."

Mass Media

Educational media about pregnancy, childbirth, and childcare now appear on television. Most of the homes in northern Louisiana have television sets; therefore, television has influenced the attitudes of these women. For instance, a 16-year-old girl said:

> I wanted my baby to be healthy. The nurse said my baby might be sick because I was so skinny. I was watching T.V. and I saw all those sick babies in the hospital with tubes in them. So I tried to eat better.

One woman, after seeing *FYI,* a television show that gives health tips, said:

> I wouldn't let my baby look at himself in the mirror because [her mother told her] it makes it hard for babies to cut teeth. Then I watched *FYI* and he said it was good for babies to see themselves in the mirror.

Availability of Resources

Although Louisiana is a rural state, a large majority of its citizens live in the cities of Shreveport or Bossier City where the combined population reaches 394,196 (Shreveport Chamber of Commerce, 1982). Therefore, blacks and whites are in contact at schools, churches, jobs, and civic activities. This provides an opportunity for ideas and beliefs to be exchanged. Facilities are closer and more available to blacks than they have been in the past. Women in the present study said that they "talked to neighbors," and "attended prenatal classes." One woman said about bathing during menstruation:

> We lived in the country. We bathed in a big washtub on the outside and it was cold. If I would have had a bathroom like I do now, I probably would have taken a bath.

Some women who lived in rural areas found health services inaccessible. These women said that mother and neighbors gave them the only advice they got. The health unit was, "too far anyway."

Developmental Level

In this study, it was found that young girls (14–17) who lived with their parents and were mothers themselves, depended more on their mothers for guidance than outside sources. This dependence seems contrary to what Erickson tells us about adolescent development. According to Erickson (1963), in adolescence, the young person is struggling to emancipate himself or herself from the authority of parents, whose own developmental tasks as parents call for sustained guidance and supervision of the not yet adult child. Erickson himself, however, pointed out that cultural traditions effect the ways in which a child develops.

WHO BUYS WHAT SYSTEM

Three kinds of clients were discovered in this study: the *corporate buyer* who buys the dominant culture health beliefs, the *cultural buyer* who buys only folk beliefs, and the *careful shopper* who buys a part of each system.

Corporate Buyer

The corporate buyer buys the dominant health care system completely. These women referred to the traditional beliefs as "superstitious" and "old wives tales." One 20-year-old woman said:

> I just told my mother that stuff was superstitious. She said if I raise my hand above my head while I'm pregnant, I'll choke the baby . . . it didn't make sense to me.

Another subject said, "I was having a hard time with my pregnancy, so I did whatever the doctors told me to." A young woman whose mother had warned her against the stretches said:

> My mother said not to let anybody hold the baby if she's menstruating. She said it would give the baby the stretches or something. [Laughs] But I didn't believe it.

Careful Shopper

The careful shopper balances between the folk health system and the dominant health system. She listens to the traditional beliefs and the dominant health care beliefs. She filters new information through her memories of past experiences, failures, and successes, and makes the decision based on a balance of the three processes, respect-fear, testing, and cultural interaction. This was evidenced by a school teacher who said:

> Mama didn't think I ought to go outside for a month after the baby came because I'd get sick. . . . I asked the nurse and she said it was all right to

go outside. None of the books said that I had to stay inside. My husband had brought my mother down to stay with me for a couple of weeks . . . so I told her that the doctor said a little fresh air every day was good for me.

This woman followed a portion of the dominant health care system in spite of the fact that her mother was staying with her.

Cultural Buyer

The third client buys no part of the dominant health care system. She is the woman who later becomes a cultural warehouse, or a conveyor of beliefs. In the study, these women were older with little formal education or very young mothers who lived in the house with an older woman. They made comments such as, "It's always worked before," and "We didn't used to depend on the doctors for every little thing." These women lived in rural areas around other people with similar beliefs and had little contact with other cultures.

CONCLUSIONS AND NURSING IMPLICATIONS

The Ethno-Market System discovered in this study of northern Louisiana black women might be used as a framework for nurses who wish to breach the gap in cross-cultural communication and teaching. The crux of this system seems to be the importance of nurses showing respect to their clients and the client's values. When the clients in this study felt that their caregivers belittled them or their cultural beliefs, they usually became what is popularly called in nursing circles, "noncompliant." It seems especially important for nurses to show respect for older black women since it is the older woman who is responsible for health teaching in most of the black families we talked with. This woman is unlikely to accept the nurse's ideas about health care, even on a *testing* basis, unless the nurse honors the older woman's beliefs. Establishing the appropriate alliances enables the *cultural buyer* to become a *careful shopper,* and integrate "scientific" remedies along with folk remedies and self-care.

The processes discovered in this study complement the findings of a previous study concerning health care beliefs of Philippine-born Americans (Stern, 1981). Findings from that study clearly indicate that nurses who showed respect for clients and their beliefs stood a better chance of bridging cultural barriers to health teaching.

It seems to us that the importance of showing respect transcends cultural boundaries. In sum, nurses may be wise to practice "health care that protects the ego system and cultural heritage . . . of all patients [of] whatever ethnic stripe" (Stern, Tilden, & Maxwell, 1980, p. 79).

REFERENCES

Bohannan, P. (1981). The ghost of Diogenes. *Science, 2,* 10, 21, 24.

Elkins, S. (1979). *Slavery: A problem in American institutional and intellectual life.* New York: Grossett & Dunlap.

Erickson, E. H. (1963). *Childhood and society.* (2nd ed.) New York: Norton. (Original version published 1950).

Frazier, F. (1939). *The Negro family in the United States.* Chicago: University of Chicago Press.

Glaser, B. G., & Strauss, A. L. (1967). *The discovery of grounded theory.* Chicago: Aldine.

Greathouse, B., & Miller, V. (1981). The black American. In A. Clark (Ed.), *Culture and childbearing,* Philadelphia: Davis.

Harrison, I., & Harrison, D. (1971/1978). The black family experience and health behavior. *Health and the Family.* New York: MacMillan.

Ladner, J. (1971). *Tomorrow's tomorrow: The black woman.* New York: Anchor.

Powers, B. (1982). The use of orthodox and black American folk medicine. *Advances in Nursing Science, 4*(3), 45.

Reeder, S., Mastrionni, L., & Martin, L. (1980). *Maternity nursing.* Philadelphia: Lippincott.

Rodgers-Rose, L. (1980). *The black woman.* Beverly Hills: Sage.

Shreveport Chamber of Commerce, Bureau of the Census, 1982.

Snow, L. (1974). Folk medical beliefs and their implications for care of patients. *Annals of Internal Medicine, 81,* 82–96.

Staples, R. (1973). *The black woman in America.* Chicago: Nelson-Hall.

Stern, P. N. (1980). Grounded theory methodology: Its uses and processes. *Image, 12*(1), 20–23.

Stern, P. N. (1981). Solving problems of cross-cultural health teaching: The Filipino childbearing family, *Image, 13*(6), 45–50.

Stern, P. N., Tilden, V. P., & Maxwell, E. K. (1980). Culturally-induced stress during childbearing: The Filipino-American experience. *Issues in Health Care of Women, 2,* 67–81.

Webb, J. (1971). Louisiana voodoo and superstitions related to health. *Health Republic, 86,* 291–301.

Williams, R. A. (1975). *Textbook of black related diseases.* New York: McGraw-Hill.

Withers, C. (1966). The folklore of a small town. *Medical Care.* New York: Wiley.

THE VIETNAMESE WOMAN: HEALTH/ILLNESS ATTITUDES AND BEHAVIORS

Mary Atchity Calhoun
St. Elizabeth Hospital, Beaumont, Texas

Vietnamese health beliefs may seem strange to western nurses. Basic to working with this or any immigrant culture is to have an understanding of and respect for cultural values. This paper presents an overview of a number of health beliefs held by a population of Vietnamese immigrants living in Texas.

There is an old Vietnamese saying that reads: "Just as the length of a road is known only by actually traveling on it, the qualities of a man are known only by living with him for a long time" (Miller, Chambers, & Aitken, 1979).

As the number of Vietnamese refugees entering the United States continues to increase, nurses are faced with the challenge of providing care to a cultural group that is very different from their own. In order to provide holistic, cultural-specific patient care, the nurse must first come to know the "qualities" of the patient in light of the cultural group to which that individual belongs.

To expedite the "coming to know" process, the qualities that will be described here are the health and illness attitudes and behaviors of Vietnamese women. Based on an exploratory study (Calhoun, 1981) and a review of the current available literature, these specific attitudes and behaviors will be discussed within the context of the broader Vietnamese culture.

CULTURAL OVERVIEW

Family

In Vietnamese society, the family is the primary source of social identity for the individual. Obligation to one's family takes priority over obligations to one's self, religion, and country. Since the family is responsible for all decisions and individual action, a person's behavior reflects shame or honor on his or her entire family (Dobbins, Lynch, Fischer, & Santopietro, 1981).

The structural unit of the traditional Vietnamese household is the extended family, usually consisting of three generations. Reflecting a longstanding tradition that males are honored and respected, the family is patriarchal in nature: the senior male is the head of the household. A Vietnamese woman lives with her husband's family after marriage, but she retains her own identity.

Within the family the division of labor is sex linked: the husband deals with matters outside of the home and the wife is responsible for the actual care of the home. Although her role in family affairs increases with time, a Vietnamese wife is expected to be dutiful and respectful toward her husband and his parents throughout the marriage.

Female immigrants to the United States are likely to remain in the home while their husbands and children attend school, get jobs, and make contacts with the outside world. The other family members gain new skills, but the Vietnamese woman tends to remain isolated within the home and grows more dependent upon her family to meet her needs.

The order of a Vietnamese person's name is important in emphasizing one's lineage. For example, Nguyen Thi Yen is a female's name with the family name written first, the middle name second, and the given name last.

Religion

One of the primary assumptions associated with the nature of life experience shared by almost all Vietnamese is that of universal order in which the processes of heaven and earth display a fundamental regularity and harmony of operation. In their basic make-up, human beings too are completely in harmony with this arranged order. The sun, moon, stars, and four seasons as well as all human relationships are controlled by natural principle (Vietnamese Resettlement Program Directorate for Southeast Texas, 1976).

The majority of Vietnamese are Buddhists, but about 10% are Catholic. Another prevalent religious influence is the philosophy of Confucius. For example, rites honoring one's ancestors are performed on feast days and on the anniversary of the death of each ancestor. Also widespread in Vietnamese society are beliefs in good and evil spirits, both animate and inanimate. Rituals are often conducted in gratitude toward or to ward off various spirits.

Family religious observances take place in the home or in the family temple, if there is one. Many Buddhists have an ancestral altar in the home set with incense, burners, and candlesticks. Altars in Catholic homes are set with religious pictures, candles, and crucifixes.

Interpersonal Relationships

The Vietnamese define social status and class distinctions more clearly than do Americans. Stressing the individual's position in a hierarchical structure, the following occupations are respected in order of increasing importance: businessman, laborer, farmer/ fisherman, scholar. A Vietnamese individual may be very reluctant to associate with another person outside of his or her social class.

A high value is placed on maintaining social harmony in interpersonal relations. This is expressed commonly through the use of tact, politeness, and gentility in dealing with others. Formality or a sense of propriety is characteristically exhibited. Because of the great value placed on social harmony, Vietnamese strive to maintain self-control. The expression of strong emotion is discouraged. The individual may smile or appear calm when he or she may actually be experiencing inner turmoil.

Most Vietnamese prefer to be approached or related to indirectly. To look another person directly in the eye shows disrespect. While handshaking is acceptable among men, women generally do not shake hands with each other or with men. Crossing one's legs, showing the bottoms of one's shoes, or pointing one's foot toward another are considered offensive and should be avoided (Gordon, Matousek, & Lang, 1980). Touching another's head without permission should also be avoided as the head is considered to be the most sacred part of the body.

HEALTH AND ILLNESS ATTITUDES AND BEHAVIORS

Explanations of Health and Illness

Health is viewed as but one facet of life in the universe, functioning as part of a unified, comprehensive scheme. In harmony with nature, the human body operates with a delicate balance between two basic opposite elements: *Am* (yin) and *Duong* (yang), or Male and Female, or Light and Dark. The *Am* and *Duong* elements also have the connotation of "Hot" and "Cold" associated with them, respectively, but these classifications have nothing to do with temperature, per se. As an example, spicy foods may be "hot," certain vegetables and bland foods "cold." The concept extends to other areas however. Viewed in this light, health is the perfect equilibrium of hot and cold elements. An excess in either direction may lead to discomfort and illness (Tran, 1980).

In addition to this metaphysical explanation for illness, the Vietnamese believe in naturalistic causes. For example, one may become sick from eating spoiled food. Lastly, it is also believed that illness can be caused by supernaturalistic entities such as gods and spirits. The punishment or illness the person experiences is viewed as the consequence of offending the god or spirit, violating a moral or religious code, or by malevolence on the part of the supernatural being.

Demonstrating the plurality of causes accepted as leading to illness, the study I conducted revealed the following results: 85% of the female respondents agreed with the statement that illness could be caused by not getting the proper exercise and not eating right; 75% agreed that sickness can be punishment for sins, and 65% agreed that many illnesses are caused by evil spirits. Seventy percent of the female subjects indicated a belief that illness results from disharmony or imbalance with the universe.

Disease Prevention and Treatment

Female respondents in my study were also asked to indicate how important certain health concepts were to them. The majority of subjects responded that good health, cleanliness, family relationships, and health teaching were of great importance. Telling someone else about your feelings was viewed as not important by 65% of the respondents.

The Vietnamese believe that one's health can be maintained by keeping a balance between the opposing forces of *Am* and *Duong*. It is also believed that illness can be prevented by offering prayers and sacrifices to various gods and spirits.

Recognizing that illness can also stem from natural causes, the majority of female subjects in my study stated that vaccinations, routine physical examinations, exercise, sleep/rest, and a balanced diet were of at least some importance to them. When asked how recently either they or their children had received an immunization, 60% responded that it had been within the last year. However, 65% had never had their eyes tested for vision and 55% had never been to a dentist or taken their children to a dentist.

Regarding hygienic practices, 70% reported that they bathed at least once a day and 90% stated that they brushed their teeth once or twice a day. Teeth lacquering is a preventive practice commonly seen in older Vietmanese women. This is a process that involves staining the teeth with a special substance that turns them black and protects them against decay.

The Vietnamese combine folk medicine and traditional practices with the latest Western scientific techniques in the treatment of illness. For example, both medicinal herbs and Western drugs are acceptable in the treatment of various illnesses, but these are carefully classified according to their properties along a scale of hot and cold effects in an effort to maintain the desired balance. Used for chills or exposure to cold, ginger is considered hot. Ginseng is thought to be a powerful panacea and is known for its cooling effects. Western medicines are thought of as hot, while Oriental herb medicines are generally considered to be cold.

Since water is looked upon as cold, a sick person generally restricts his or her fluid intake to avoid creating more of an imbalance. External use of water is also avoided during illness for the same reason. A Vietnamese patient may be reluctant to bathe or shower.

Aspects of Vietnamese folk medicine include rice alcohol for toothaches and rhinoceros horn to lower fever. Other medicinal substances include deer antler, dried bumblebees, orange peel, and mint (Tao-Kim-Hai, 1965). Many Vietnamese use Tiger Balm (an oil or ointment with a menthol base) to fight a cold, settle the stomach, or relieve a headache. It can be rubbed under the nose, on the stomach, or on the forehead.

The practice of CaoGaó ("rubbing out the wind") is very commonly used for the treatment of minor ailments (Golden & Duster, 1977). It consists of forcefully rubbing particular areas of the forehead, base of the nose, neck, chest, and back with either a coin or the fingers. If done properly, this procedure will leave long lines of continuous dark bruises on the skin.

Local practitioners are common in Vietnam and they provide such treatments as acupuncture, scarification at strategic points on the skin, suction with small tubes or hot cups, and moxibustion. The last of these involves burning a soft substance, moxa on the skin.

Seventy percent of the female subjects in my study indicated that they used home remedies when sick. Examples of these included Tiger Balm with the use of a coin for headaches, stomachaches, sinus problems, and dizziness, and pinching of the neck and forehead for headaches. Lastly, taking a steam bath with a menthol-based oil was reportedly used for colds.

Western medications, especially antibiotics, are acceptable to the Vietnamese in the treatment of illness. It is a common practice in

Vietnam to self-medicate because many drugs (such as antibiotics) are dispensed without a prescription by pharmacies there.

Loss of blood from any route is greatly feared (Devitt, 1966) and the Vietnamese individual may even refuse to have his or her blood drawn for lab tests. Because of a fear of mutilation, there is also a great resistance to surgery, unless as a last resort. Hospitalization is also viewed as a last resort and is acceptable only in cases of emergency or when everything else has failed. Prayers and offerings may be made at the local temple in an effort to appease an evil spirit or god believed to have caused an illness.

Nutrition

The normal daily caloric intake for a Vietnamese individual is approximately two thirds that of an average American because of the Oriental's smaller size (Dobbins, Lynch, & Fischer, 1980). Rice is the staple food in the diet and it provides up to 80% of the calories consumed daily (U.S. Department of Agriculture Food and Nutrition Service, 1980). Other foods commonly eaten include noodle soup, green vegetables, small amounts of meat (particularly pork and chicken), and fish. When available, bananas, mangos, papayas, oranges, coconuts, and pineapples are preferred fruits. Garlic, black pepper, onions, soy sauce, and fish sauce (nuoc mam) are used in preparing food. In my study, rice, fish/shellfish, green vegetables, and pork were the foods reported as most commonly eaten. Water and tea were the beverages reported as most frequently consumed.

The daily meal pattern consists of three meals and optional snacks. Meals are served communal style and may be eaten with chopsticks. Stir-frying, roasting, boiling, and steaming are preferred methods of cooking. Fat content in the diet is small.

Because many adult Vietnamese have a lactase deficiency, dairy products are generally avoided. Small amounts of sweetened condensed milk are tolerated though and sometimes used in coffee.

Extreme diets or those that include too much of hot or cold foods are avoided because of the belief in balancing the hot and cold elements. Ninety percent of the female respondents interviewed in my study indicated that they believed illness could be prevented by a balanced diet.

Most spices, sweets, candies, fish sauce, peppers, and onions are considered hot. Vegetables, fruits, rice, flour, meats, fish, and potatoes are considered cold. Tea is cold while coffee is hot. Water is cold but ice is considered to be hot. Cold foods can become hot with the addition of hot foods.

One aim of treatment during illness is to balance the diet very carefully according to the hot and cold theory. Fifty-five percent of the females interviewed indicated that certain foods were consumed in greater quantity during illness such as a light rice gruel (chao) mixed with sugar or sweetened condensed milk, and a few pieces of salty pork cooked with fish sauce. Until the patient is recuperating, fresh vegetables and fruits are usually avoided as they are considered too cold. Fresh meats are reintroduced slowly.

The Vietnamese do not generally consume a great deal of alcohol except for a rice wine that is commonly available. None of the females I interviewed admitted to drinking alcoholic beverages. Smoking is not widely practiced and even then, it is less acceptable for women than men: 95% of the female subjects stated that they did not smoke. Chewing betel leaves (chau) is a practice of older Vietnamese women and is believed to have a narcotic effect on diseased gums.

Housing Conditions

Because of the "extended" nature of the Vietnamese family, it is not uncommon for three to four generations to live together in one house. This has become a matter of necessity also for many Vietnamese refugees due to the financial problems of resettlement and aggravated housing conditions. It was commonly reported by the women in my study that there might be six to ten people living in only three- and four-room dwellings.

Child-Bearing and Child-Rearing

The Vietnamese female tends to be shy and may resist disrobing when examination is required. She may refuse to have a pelvic examination. Sexuality is not readily discussed and the Vietnamese female may even be reluctant to discuss her menstrual periods. For obstetrical and gynecological matters, she usually feels more comfortable with a female doctor or midwife (Chung, 1977).

In rural areas of Vietnam a woman very commonly has her baby at home with the services of a midwife. She may not be accustomed to prenatal checkups. Those living in Vietnamese cities and women immigrating to the United States are more familiar with prenatal examinations and delivery by a doctor in a hospital. Seventy-five percent of the females I interviewed indicated that they thought the monthly examinations were important; 95% indicated that they would go to a hospital to have a baby, and 70% would request the services of a doctor.

Although pregnancy is seen as a normal or natural process, the Vietnamese have certain taboos and follow special customs during this time. For example, the subjects in my study explained that they ate more noodles, sweets, sour foods, and fruits such as mangos. Foods that were avoided during the pregnancy included salty items, rice, and fish. Many consider it taboo to attend weddings and funerals while pregnant (Hollingsworth, Brown, & Brooten, 1980). Regarding activity during pregnancy, 65% of the women in my study agreed that a woman should change her work habits when pregnant.

Once in labor the Vietnamese female will maintain the self-control that is typical of the culture as a whole; she may even smile continuously. Her labor period is generally short and there may not be much advance warning of her impending delivery. She may prefer to walk around during labor and choose to deliver the baby in a squatting position.

Vietnamese women believe that a great deal of body heat is lost during the delivery process. Consequently cold foods and drinks are avoided after delivery. Fifty-five percent of the women in my study indicated that they consumed less cold water, raw vegetables, and fruit in the postpartum period. Seventy-five percent reported eating more eggs, spicy and salty foods, and boiled cabbage during this time. A sort of stew made of rice, pork, and fish sauce was described as popular to restore strength.

Early ambulation and strenuous activity are avoided in the postpartum period because they are believed to hinder one's internal organs from returning to their normal position. Fifty-five percent of the women I interviewed indicated that they would stay in bed approximately one month after delivery. A new mother may also refuse to bathe or shampoo her hair for a month or so as she fears that too much water applied externally and exposure to cold air may cause loss of nutrients and energy through the skin (Stringfello, 1978). She may be persuaded however, to take a sponge bath.

New mothers from rural areas of Vietnam generally breastfeed their infants while those from the city or those who hold jobs prefer to bottle-feed. Many believe that it is more acceptable in the United States to bottle-feed. The women in my study were equally divided on the subject. Those preferring to breastfeed stated that on the average, they would nurse a child for $1-1\frac{1}{2}$ years.

A newborn is often dressed in old clothes and it is considered taboo to praise the child. These customs prevail to prevent jealous spirits from stealing the infant. A new mother will also avoid cutting the child's hair and nails to avoid causing illness.

Introducing solid foods other than rice gruel to the infant's diet is generally delayed until the child is a year old. Sixty percent of the subjects in my study stated that they would wait until the child was at least 6 months old before introducing any solids at all.

The Vietnamese tend to be more relaxed in their attitude toward toilet-training. Little effort is put into formally training the child: one learns toilet habits by imitating an older child. Often times a toddler or preschooler goes without diapers or underpants.

Vietnamese children tend to be shy and are generally well-behaved. Discipline consists of speaking to a child in a quiet, controlled manner. Spanking or slapping a child's hands is not usually practiced. However, as a means of punishment, having a child kneel and face the wall quietly was reportedly practiced by 45% of the subjects I interviewed. As a child gets older, parents expect their children to follow their guidance without argument or questioning.

Mental Illness

Although the Vietnamese embrace both the organic model and the hot-cold theory as possibly playing roles in mental illness, the most widely accepted explanation is that it is the result of a supernatural event. A mental condition is stigmatizing to both an individual and the family because mental illness is believed to result from offending a god or demon or committing a sin. An individual with a mental condition can jeopardize the ability of other family members to find marriage partners. For this reason, a family will try to protect and hide a mentally ill person from the public. Fifty-five percent of the women I interviewed stated that a person having mental problems was a disgrace to his or her family.

Since physical complaints are more acceptable than those of an emotional nature, the individual with an emotional problem will tend to somatize it. The cultural inhibition against expressing one's negative feelings is so effective that even in psychotic episodes, the Vietnamese individual is rarely violent.

The family will take responsibility for the welfare of a mentally ill individual in the home as long as his or her behavior can be con-trolled or tolerated. If therapy or help is sought for this person, it is with the greatest discretion, and sometimes after a dangerously long delay.

Death and Mourning

Many Vietnamese would prefer to die at home rather than in the hospital, the belief being that a person who dies outside the home becomes a wandering soul with no place to rest. Sixty percent of the women in my study responded that if someone in their family was dying they would not want that person to be told; 95% stated that they would want a priest or minister with them when they died, and 95% indicated that they believed in life after death.

The mourning period for a deceased person is accompanied by certain practices. For example, when one's parent dies, a child must wait 3 years before marrying, as must a woman when her husband dies. A husband must wait 1 year to remarry when his wife dies. In mourning, all white clothes are worn for 14 days; after that, men wear black arm bands and women wear white head bands. Because the family is viewed as a continuous lineage in time, ancestors are commonly worshipped and honored for the protection and powers they are believed to bestow on the living. The anniversary date of a person's death is celebrated yearly, the eldest son taking responsibility for the ancestor worship.

Role of the Patient, Family, and Physician

An individual who is ill will not readily complain of pain or discomfort since Vietnamese culture idealizes stoicism and views endurance as an indicator of strong character. A person may delay seeking attention for a disease until it is in the advanced stages. During illness, the Vietnamese individual is allowed to be dependent on his or her family and receives a great deal of attention and care.

The female is usually the chief health care provider in the family or takes the most responsibility for the health of the rest of the family (Gallow, Edwards, & Vessey, 1980). This was confirmed in my study: 70% of the female subjects cited themselves as the chief health care giver. Family members will stay with the patient in the hospital and bring nourishing foods from home. Sixty-five percent of the women I interviewed stated that the would want someone to stay with them in the hospital if they were sick.

Health care professionals are generally expected to assume a highly authoritative role in the care of a Vietnamese patient (Santopietro, 1980). Ninety percent of the female subjects agreed with the statement that they could only do what their doctors tell them to do. Ninety-five percent felt that for most kinds of illnesses, a doctor could help them the most; 85% felt that the drugs doctors prescribe are better than home remedies. In general, a positive attitude toward doctors and nurses was conveyed by the majority of female respondents.

CONCLUSION

Transcultural nursing is, first of all, a "coming to know" process. As a nurse begins to learn and understand the health and illness attitudes and behaviors of those belonging to immigrant cultures (don't we all?), the nurse experiences her or his own individualized reactions based on the teaching and beliefs of her or his own culture. One might, for instance, agree that the Vietnamese practice of breastfeeding infants for $1\frac{1}{2}$-2 years is preferable for infant nutrition and facilitates maternal-infant bonding; but reject the idea that a month of bed rest is necessary for organs to return to their normal position. Where folk beliefs aid in keeping ego integrity intact and do not interfere with normal physical or psychological well-being, professionals would be well advised to show them due respect. A friendly, interested approach would seem to enhance an atmosphere of mutual trust. This mutual trust may encourage the communication of other folk beliefs or practices that might not be in the interest of optimum health maintenance. A culturally sensitive nurse would then be able to strategize her approaches to health care and teaching so that ego structure is not threatened and trust is kept intact. Offensive behaviors could be avoided to preserve the nurse-client relationship. New methods of health care teaching could be introduced as acceptable alternatives while feedback is elicited in order to modify or reintroduce new ideas. Where issues are discovered that are nonnegotiable, the right of the client to decide must be upheld.

REFERENCES

Calhoun, M. A. (1981). *Vietnamese health/illness attitudes and behaviors.* Unpublished master's thesis, University of Texas, Galveston.

Chung, H. J. (1977, March). Understanding the Oriental maternity patient. *Nursing Clinics of North America, 12,* 67–75.

Devitt, H. (1966, December). Nursing in a Vietnamese village. *Nursing Outlook, 14,* 46–49.

Dobbins, E., Lynch, B., & Fischer, D. (1980, September). Translating the Indochinese diet into English. *RN, 43,* 79.

Dobbins, E., Lynch, B., Fischer, D., & Santopietro, M. C. S. (1981, January). A beginner's guide to Vietnamese culture. *RN, 44,* 44–45.

Gallo, A., Edwards, J., & Vessey, J. (1980, December). Little refugees with big needs. *RN, 43,* 45–48.

Golden, S., & Duster, M. (1977, October). Hazards of misdiagnosis due to Vietnamese folk medicine. *Clinical Pediatrics,* pp. 949–950.

Gordon, V., Matousek, I., & Lang, T. (1980, November). Southeast Asian refugees: Life in America. *American Journal of Nursing, 80,* 2031–2036.

Hollingsworth, A., Brown, L., & Brooten, D. (1980, November). The refugees and childbearing: What to expect. *RN, 43,* 45–48.

Miller, B., Chambers, E., & Aitken, W. (Eds.). (1979). *Indochinese adjustment service manual and directory.* Commonwealth of Pennsylvania, Department of Public Welfare, p. 16.

Santopietro, M. C. S., & Lynch, B. (1980, October). What's behind the 'inscrutable' mask? *RN, 43,* 55–61.

Stringfellow, L. (1978). The Vietnamese. In A. Clark (Ed.), *Culture, Childbearing, Health Professionals.* Philadelphia: Davis.

Tao-Kim-Hai, A. (1965). Orientals are stoic. In J. Skipper & R. Leonard (Eds.), *Social Interaction and Patient Care.* Philadelphia: Lippincott.

Tran, M. T. (1980). *Indochinese patients.* Washington, DC: Action for Southeast Asians.

U.S. Department of Agriculture Food and Nutrition Service. (1980, September). *Southeast Asian American Food Habits.* FNS-225.

Vietnamese Resettlement Program Directorate for Southeast Texas. (1976). *A Guide to Working with Vietnamese Refugees.* Christian Life Center, Beaumont, Texas.

IDEOLOGY AND ILLNESS EXPERIENCES OF WOMEN IN GUATEMALA

Joyceen S. Boyle, RN, PhD
University of Utah, Salt Lake City, Utah

The position of women in the society of a Guatemalian *colonia* influences both self-care and the care given them. The description of this cultural group provides universal meaning regarding women's health and social position.

Women in Latin American countries, as in much of the world today, live in class-based societies where men hold the dominant positions of power and economic control. However, the degree of power held by women varies greatly in relation to one another and to men, depending upon such variables as class, the degree of stratification in the society, and conditions of political instability, social revolution, or rapid capitalization.

The study of the incorporation of sexual ideologies in religious systems and the role of ideology in stating the qualities and capabilities of men and women and in perpetuating these beliefs through time is a major concern in the study of women. Improvements in the general economic conditions and changes in legal and health care systems do not necessarily involve improved conditions for women and much of the resistance to alter the bases of sexual inequality rests in ideological and religious beliefs (Beck & Keddie, 1978, p. 30). While the role of ideology is not a sufficient explanation for the universality of women's subordination, ideologies have tended to legitimize and provide credence for the lower status of women. Cultural ideologies impinge upon women and are used to keep women in their place. How belief systems might influence

This study was supported in part by National Research Service Award Grant 1F31-NU-05115-01, Department of Health, Education and Welfare, Health Resources Administration, Division of Nursing.

The original version of this paper was presented at the Eighth Annual Conference of the Transcultural Nursing Society and is included in the Conference Proceedings.

health and illness experiences requires further analysis of particular ideologies in relation to women's illness experiences. This paper uses a theoretical frame of reference that organizes observations about manifestations of behavior and the etiology of illness. This framework suggests a nursing paradigm for analyzing women's health problems that has implications for nursing roles in the prevention of illness and in the maintenance of health. The practice of nursing requires knowledge of human relationships and the effects of sociocultural factors associated with both health and illness. The behavior of individuals under circumstances over which they have little or no control gives pertinent data for the study of human behavior and suggests possibilities for the application of concepts used in nursing.

The data presented in this paper were collected in an urban area in the central highlands of western Guatemala. Examples are drawn from a purposive sample of 134 individuals that was almost equally divided by sex (66 females and 68 males) and varied by age. Fifty-seven percent of the population were 15 years of age or older. The sample consisted of Cakchiquel Indians living in 22 extended households within the geographical boundaries of a small *colonia.* * For the most part, sample members (both men and women) were unskilled or semiskilled workers, lacking both job security and income stability.

The study was carried out during a 13-month fieldwork experience. Participant observation and interviews were used to obtain information regarding ideological systems and health and illness behaviors. Behaviors were observed and recorded; inferences regarding beliefs that influenced behavior were determined with assistance from the informants in the study. During the course of the study, households were followed for a 4-week period using a family health calendar recording (FHCR) and focused interviews to elicit data regarding illness experiences and associated belief systems.

This paper specifically examines the emotionally related illness experiences of women within a broader analysis that integrates the social and ideological components of sexual asymmetry. It will be argued that for these Guatemalan Indian women, traditional relations and attitudes derived from sexual and religious interpretations of reality were manifested in women's illness experiences.

WOMEN'S ROLES AND OCCUPATIONS

Women in the colonia are socialized early in life in roles that are strictly divided along sexual lines. At the age of four or five years,

---

*In Guatemala, a *colonia* is a politically defined urban settlement.

young girls begin to learn household tasks by sharing domestic responsibilities with their mothers or older sisters. Young boys may help carry water, but they have more freedom to play in the streets, tease their sisters, and generally come and go as they please. It is not uncommon to see deference given to sons by mothers and sisters.

Young girls are allowed the greatest freedom in terms of physical activities prior to puberty; at age 10 or 12 years their outside activities are more restricted, and they are kept closer to the home. Teenage girls may participate in social activities, but it is usually done in conjunction with other girls or family members. Girls who do not behave "appropriately" are considered fair game for men. Both men and women in the colonia equate the feminist movement in the United States with sexual promiscuity.

Gossip and displays of envy such as resentfulness of advantages enjoyed by others are common means of social control to influence the behavior of young women who transgress community norms. There is little support of women by other women. This lack of mutual support manifests itself in lack of empathy and understanding between women, quarreling, bickering, and the absence of trust.

Young girls in the colonia complete an average of 6 years of schooling after which they primarily spend the next few years helping their mothers with the household responsibilities; a few may take jobs as domestic servants. Marriage occurs at a relatively young age in the colonia, usually during the late teens for the girl and early twenties for the boy. Not all marriages are formalized by legal sanction; of the 22 households in the sample, only 41% of the heads of households had been legally married.

After marriage many young women of the colonia seek full-time employment outside of the home. Their work roles are extensions of their domestic responsibilities; they are employed as domestic servants, cleaning women, food vendors in the market, and occasionally as cooks or waitresses in food establishments. Many women earn additional income from cooking and selling foodstuffs, raising pigs or chickens, selling eggs, sewing, and collecting tin cans and bottles for resale. These activities represent an important source of added income and cash reserve to the meager financial resources of the family.

Routine observations of daily living activities indicated that all women work, often from early childhood, even though they may not be formally employed. Beck and Keddie (1978, p. 3) stated that women's activities usually are not regarded as work because they are not directly compensated. A man whose occupation is that of an unskilled construction worker is viewed as a legitimate worker, while his wife, who arises at 4 a.m. to carry water and wash clothes by hand, raises and tends domestic animals, grinds corn by hand, produces handicrafts for the market, cleans house, gives birth and raises children, and perhaps sells her hand-made tortillas in the streets during the afternoons and evenings often is viewed as economically inactive, even though her tasks are crucial to the maintenace of the family and society. Nearly all adult women in the colonia earned $20–$30 per month from various enterprises such as selling eggs, food, or handicrafts. Analysis of routine activities in the colonia indicated that women, on the average, worked longer hours than did the men and received little in wages. Even women with full-time employment as domestics seldom received more than the equivalent of $20–$30 per month. Men's wages, although higher than those of women, were minimal also. The male heads of households averaged only $67 per month.

Women's work, whether in the home or a more formal setting, is not valued as highly as that of men. Women's status and position in the workplace is seen as merely an extension of domestic roles. When men were asked what activities or tasks were the responsibility of women, one man replied, "those tasks that can be done sitting down" and "women just cook." Most men said very emphatically that cooking, washing clothes, and dishes were "women's work" and that they would never do it. There was considerable peer pressure among men that reinforced such beliefs and behavior. A man who washed clothes or dishes or otherwise assisted his wife with such tasks was ridiculed as being "less than a man" or "good for nothing else."

There seemed to be no particular negative feelings on the part of men if their wives or daughters were gainfully employed outside of the home. This tolerant attitude toward employment of females may have been influenced by a number of factors. Economic necessity is forcing many women to seek employment, especially in areas that are undergoing urbanization and capitalization expansion. Then, too, Indian women have always been involved in the market systems of Guatemala. They are able to take their children with them, and thus have circumvented this particular barrier to working outside of the home.

It is important to reiterate that a working wife does not affect the male role significantly. Women, whether formally employed or not, are still responsible for all domestic tasks, including the care of children and all household responsibilities. Working outside the home is something a woman does in addition to other role-prescribed responsibilities.

Women in the sample indicated that they enjoy the opportunity to work outside the home. In a society that still restricts the role of women by limiting their mobility outside of the household, a job provides a socially approved reason for women to leave the confines of the home. In addition, women said that they wanted to have a little money of their own and not be dependent upon their husbands.

STRUCTURE OF MALE–FEMALE RELATIONSHIPS

Among the residents of the colonia there are a number of traditional beliefs that relate to the ascribed qualities or characteristics of men and women. These beliefs are used to explain or justify the "natural" differences between the sexes. Women, of course, are viewed as being inherently weaker than men. It is believed that women are not able to work as hard as men, and by virtue of this weakness cannot withstand heat, cold, exhaustion, and other adversities as well as men. Childbirth and menstruation render women weak and special precautions must be taken during these periods for extra protection. Such beliefs establish men as the "protectors" of women by virtue of "his strength" and "her weakness." This contributes to a belief in male superiority and reinforces the notion that tough, domineering men should be valued by women because such men are "naturally" better able to take care of women. The reliance on men for care and protection places women in dependent positions, which often results in some measure of male control and dominance.

The belief that man is superior to women also dominates male-female relationships. This cultural tradition of male dominance is usually referred to as *machismo.* It is described by O'Kelly (1980) as a "cult of virility" (p. 199). Stevens (1973) states that machismo is an "exaggerated aggressiveness and intransigence in male-to-male interpersonal relationships and arrogance and sexual aggression in male-to-female relationships" (p. 90). Originally introduced into the New World by the Spanish conquistadores, machismo is more evident in the *Ladino* or non-Indian population of Guatemala. However, the data in this study indicate that the colonial legacy of machismo has affected urban-based indigenous communities to some extent; it is more apparent in younger males than in the older ones.

Women's virginity prior to marriage is highly valued as is chaste and modest conduct after marriage. Parents try hard to restrict their daughters' freedom, and in particular, to keep them from being alone with men. Dating is rare in the colonia. On the other hand, parents do not feel the same obligation to keep their sons sheltered and away from sexual experimentation. If a woman agrees to have sex with a man, it is her fault and not his. Men are naturally expected to pursue sex whenever the opportunity arises.

In the extreme, it is assumed that females cannot control themselves sexually. If someone is to be reproached, it is the woman who should not have put herself in a situation where she could provoke the desire of a man. Comradeship or friendship among men and women is suspect; all verbal communication and all physical approaches take on a sexual connotation and are open to suspicion. For a woman in the street to laugh, for example, is an amorous call; to meet a man's eyes with hers is a solicitation. For a woman to be alone with a man presupposes that sex will occur because women are unable to control their sexual impulses.

The ideology to which men adhere and to some extent women also, expresses the belief that women are impressionable, lacking in judgment, and treacherous, and must, therefore, be controlled. Women are thought of as temptresses, without moral sense or responsibility. While these are statements in the extreme to make a point, the underlying ideology is clear. Women are not to be trusted because of their sexuality. Men need to be cautious of women because, although they are weaker and inferior to men, they may use their sexuality to exert influence or control men. With such beliefs, there is local folklore relating to the use of menstrual blood to "control" or "subdue" men. For example, a small amount of menstrual blood on a cloth or napkin placed by a woman under a bed where a man is sleeping will render him under her power. A bit of menstrual blood in *te' de Jamaica* (a red-colored tea) will make the man who drinks it unable to resist the sexual advances of the woman who prepared the tea.

The strict separation of marital roles in many Latin societies goes beyond the division of labor to encompass leisure, friendship, and affective roles. There is little show of emotion or affection between husband and wife in the marital relationships observed in the colonia. Many men display stronger emotional attachments to their male friends, while women direct their affective lives to their children. As a general rule, the bonding between mothers and sons appears stronger than between mother and daughters.

The women's role is one of subordination characterized by a great deal of tolerance and patience. Women grow up taking care of men, waiting on their needs and occasionally submitting to ill treatment, callousness, and neglect with stoic patience and resignation. When speaking of men's behavior such as drinking, refusing to provide money for their families, or spending all of their free time with their male friends or other women, the women said,

"That's the way it is. It is always the women and children who suffer, not the men."

The male role is most commonly dominant, often displayed through wife abuse, excessive drinking, and occasional failure to provide money for household expense. Not all of the men in the colonia drank to excess, but a large portion of them did. Sixty-four percent of the households in the sample reported a family member (always male) who frequently drank excessively, becoming abusive or threatening with his spouse. Women in the colonia tend to develop resilient personalities and learn early in life to become resourceful through enduring situations. Women do endure and survive some rather difficult times, but they do not necessarily remain isolated or passive. Often, women berated their husbands publicly and forcefully for their excessive drinking behavior or failure to provide for their families, and many suffered public beatings for this audacity.

It was believed by women that the "best" marriages were those where the husband did not drink. These marriages were described as "tranquil" and "happy." Women said "bad" marriages were those in which the husband: 1) did not give his wife money for food and household expenses, 2) had other women, and 3) drank frequently and was abusive. The unfortunate woman who had a husband with all of these qualities was greatly pitied by her kin and neighbors, and it was said that she had "bad luck." It should be noted that for these economically marginal women, financial security was the most important element in a marriage. As long as the husband supported the family, almost any behavior, including infidelity, would be tolerated. I was not aware of any married woman who participated in extramarital affairs. On the other hand, the colonia gossip indicated that a number of men in the sample and within the larger population of the colonia "had other women."

Women have few alternatives other than staying with their husbands. Because they lack economic skills, they believe that life is easier with a husband who gives them money some of the time than life as a single woman trying to support a family. Divorce is not considered as an option. Both men and women reported that a divorced woman could never remarry because "no man would have her." However, a divorced man could remarry without social stigma. Since under Guatemalan law, a woman's consent is necessary prior to a divorce, women said that they would never consent if their husband wanted a divorce. A woman would never be able to remarry anyway, so why allow the husband freedom to marry again? A woman who has separated from her husband could live with another man, and many of them chose to do so because economically they were unable to support themselves or their children. Residents of the colonia reported that often stepchildren were not readily accepted by the stepfather. Informants indicated that men prefer women who have not been married and who have not had children by another man. Occasionally, men left their families, lived with other women, and fathered other children. Informants reported that such men almost never provided financial support to their first families, although they might give a little money to their children when they encountered them in the streets.

RELIGIOUS IDEOLOGY AND SEXUAL ASYMMETRY

The Spanish conquest of Guatemala introduced agrarian, political, and sociocultural reforms. These changes included much more subordinate and oppressive roles for women (O'Kelly, 1980, p. 198). There has been extensive documentation (Adams, 1970; De La Fuente, 1967; & Beals, 1952) of the oppression and exploitation of the Indian population. The early Spaniards considered non-Europeans as inferior and native females were ranked below native men.

The Spaniards also imposed the Catholic religion on the defeated Indian population. Spanish Catholicism embodied negative views of women and supported male dominance. O'Kelly (1980) suggests that "the Church supported the division of women into the good, asexual, devoted mother figure of the Virgin Mary and the bad, seductive Eve figure" (p. 198). According to Stevens (1973), the other face of machismo is "the cultural ideal of *marianismo* or the cult of spiritual superiority of women . . . women are semidivine, morally superior to, and spiritually stronger than men" (p. 91). Stevens suggests that the Virgin Mary is the ideal role model, and women are supposed to be self-sacrificing, submissive, patient, and long suffering. Of course, not all women conform to the stereotype of marianismo. The alternative model is that of the "bad" woman who flaunts the norms and persists in enjoying herself.

The Protestant women in the sample are influenced by the norms and dictates of fundamental religions which have been particularly successful in Guatemala in converting members of the lower economic classes. These sects have attempted to impose an 18th century Victorian moralism upon their members. They continue to reinforce a subordinate gender role for women and the ideology of women's place in the home. For example, Protestant informants reported that it is "sinful" to wear makeup, to cut one's hair, to wear sleeveless dresses or pants, to drink liquor, or to dance. However, despite pressure to conform, many women deviate from these religious ideals to varying degrees.

The data in this study indicate this population of urban Indians are experiencing numerous sociocultural changes and certain forms of traditional sexual discrimination still exist. While the women in the sample do not necessarily represent the subservient, dependent, apolitical, homebound model of the stereotyped Latin women, there are many similarities. Their general view of life was expressed by one of the women who said, "Like mama, I live mainly for my family. I try to be a good wife and a good mother, but sometimes life is very hard." In general it was accepted as a basic premise of their marital relationships that their lives should be arranged to accommodate their husband's needs and desires.

It can be argued that the nominally poor Indian women in the sample are among the most powerless segment of the society. Not only do they suffer from both class and caste discrimination, but they are forced to contend with sexual inequality as well. This pattern of sexual asymmetry which the foregoing discussion has brought into focus is clearly reflected in the ideological subsystem of the culture. This is not to deny the reality of women's covert power. Power relations are not static, but are subject to patterned changes, and female power, like male authority, is a social reality. The point to be stressed is that when a woman in the colonia chooses to manipulate events to her advantage, her efforts are subject to cultural constraints imposed by the limits of her specific situation. These boundary conditions define the extent of her accomplishments and choice may be curtailed by the lack of viable alternatives.

In a situation of poverty and marginality, the standards and role models of the larger society often are irrelevant to the daily life of people even though they may be embraced on a verbal level. The conflict between the real and the ideal world of women requires a constant negotiation of reality. The system does not function smoothly; the role of women appears in particular to be composed of parts that are scarcely compatible.

It can be hypothesized that the conflicts originating from ideological interpretations of reality are made manifest in the illness experiences of women. The sick role offers a temporary modification of status or an opportunity to behave in a manner that would otherwise not be tolerated. An examination of illness experiences can be used to further explore the relation between sex roles and illness. Such an analysis can serve as a probe into social life and as an index of sex status.

DIFFERENTIAL INCIDENCE OF ILLNESS

A family health calendar recording (FHCR) was used to collect the data presented in this portion of the paper. The FHCR involved each household reporting illness incidents that occurred during a selected 4-week period. The investigator contacted each household every other day and recorded all information on the FHCR. Family members were asked to report the name of the person ill, the symptoms encountered, measures taken for alleviation of symptoms, and ascribed causation. Informants described symptoms in general symptomatic terms. The symptoms were placed into six broad general categories. The categories were respiratory, gastrointestinal, emotional, problems of the lower extremities, headaches, and other. Ill persons or family members provided information that facilitated the classification of symptoms. In particular, care was taken to classify emotionally related illnesses according to causation beliefs that were elicited from the informants. Conditions such as "stomachache," "headache," or "anger" were classified as emotionally related illnesses only when the ill person reported they were caused by "nerves" (*por los nervios*). Further questions explored the precipitating factors or events that were perceived by informants as triggering the illness symptom.

Table 1 shows that the members of the sample reported a total of 135 identifiable symptoms during this 4-week period. The data indicate that three-fourths of the women (77.4%), one-fourth of the men (24.3%), and less than half (43.3%) of the children reported illness incidents. Table 2 shows that women experienced more problems of the lower extremities, more headaches, more respiratory

Table 1. Frequency and Distribution of Family Members ($N = 132$)
Reporting Illness Incidents ($N = 135$)

	Sample members					
	Women		Men		Children[*]	
Respondents	N	%	N	%	N	%
Total respondents	31	23.5	41	31.1	60	45.4
Persons reporting illness	24	77.4	10	24.3	26	43.3
Incidents of illness	54	40.0	14	10.4	67	49.6

[*]All persons below the age of 18 years.

**Table 2. Symptoms of Illness (N = 135) Reported
by Men, Women, and Children (N = 132)**

Symptoms by category	Men (N)	Women (N)	Children (N)
Respiratory	5	9	35
Gastrointestinal and abdominal conditions	3	9	19
Emotional	1	13	
Problems of lower extremities		7	2
Headaches (nonemotional)		4	1
Other	4	11	12
Total	13	53	69

and gastrointestinal symptoms, more emotionally related problems, and higher number of other illnesses than did men.

Table 3 shows the type of emotionally related symptoms that accounted for 10.3% of the total number of illness incidents reported by the sample. As previously mentioned, emotionally derived illnesses were classified on the basis of the information supplied by the informants. All of the emotional upsets, except the one case of anger (*enojado*) were reported as occurring in women. The one case of anger in a male was reported by the man's wife, mother, and sister who complained that he was angry, abusive, and causing family disturbances. It is possible that this man would not have self-reported his anger as a symptom of illness. As a result of his behavior, female

**Table 3. Symptoms of Emotional Illness (N = 135) Reported
by the Sample (N = 132) During a One-Month Period**

Symptoms by category	Frequency reported
Cólera (headache, stomachache, and vomiting)	1
Worry, anxiety	2
Anger	1
Upset, crying	1
Depression	1
Stomachache	1
Headache	7
Total	14

family members said that they were experiencing physical abuse, headaches, stomachaches, and depression.

The differential incidence of illnesses in the sample indicate that during this 4-week period women tended to experience all types of illness and, in particular, emotional difficulties far more frequently than did men. In view of women's position of relative powerlessness and the greater restrictions imposed on them as a group, it was hypothesized that women in particular would be more likely to experience illness symptoms. Data collected by use of the FHCR lends support to the above hypothesis.

During the course of the study, field notes indicated that women and/or children primarily tended to suffer from folk illnesses. *Bilis,* believed to be caused by strong emotions of passion, anger, fright, or extreme sadness, was the most frequently reported folk illness by females. *Cólera,* which is believed caused by anger or other emotional upsets, is another term used interchangeably with bilis. Cólera is believed to be precipitated by quarreling, and in its extreme form can lead to a *desrame* or stroke.

In this society, women are viewed as quintessentially vulnerable and full of self-destructive whims, irrational behavior, innate weaknesses, and are not to be trusted. The notion that illnesses expressed the character was invariably extended to assert that the character caused the disease. This can be illustrated by a closer examination of the episode of cólera or bilis, the one incident of folk illness reported during the 4-week FHCR.

Roberto, a 22-year-old male, returned home at 2 a.m. after a long evening of drinking and partying with male companions. When his wife inquired as to his whereabouts for the past few hours, he became angry and struck her several times. His mother, awakened by the quarreling, attempted to intervene. Roberto shoved her roughly aside telling her to mind her own business. The next morning, the female informants stated that Roberto was still angry and verbally abusive and that his anger was causing illness symptoms in the household members. When asked about the causes of Roberto's anger, his sister explained that it had been caused by his drinking and the influence of the "bad" women (*mujeres malas*) that he associated with during such late hours. His mother, suffering from cólera, complained of a severe headache, a stomachache, and vomiting; she remained in bed throughout the day. The wife, in addition to a black eye, facial lacerations and bruises, was upset and crying and complained of depression, anxiety, and a stomachache. The sister, too, complained of worry, depression, and a headache. When these three women were asked about the underlying causes of their illnesses, they attributed their symptoms to women being weaker, and not able to tolerate strong emotions and upsets as well as males. In addition, the mother and sister said the incident would not have happened if the wife had not started the quarrel. They said "It's none of her business what Roberto does or where he goes. She shouldn't have bothered him and pestered him with questions."

SUMMARY AND CONCLUSIONS

The data suggest that emotionally-related illness occurs more frequently in female members of the sample because cultural traditions dictate a more circumscribed role for women. Ideological and religious beliefs do not sanction strong expressions of emotions or feelings on the part of women. Men can take out their frustrations by beating up a friend or a wife, or by getting drunk, which women cannot do. Among members of the sample, alcohol indulgence and spouse abuse were common male practices while bilis and emotionally related illness occurred in the female population.

The data cited in the foregoing analysis indicate that the incidence of reported emotional illness is associated with culturally stipulated role behavior and is directly related to the subservient status of women. The point to be stressed is that while emotional conditions and their associated physical symptoms offer a legitimate channel for temporary relief, they do not result in a permanent modification of status. Strategies of indirect control, including illness, are subject to the confines of culture and situational restraints.

Women's health care in every society is a reflection of the total culture. Health and illness are related to the social organization, the political system, and the religious system as much as they are to the medical system of a particular society. Different sociohistorical contexts, perceptions of experiences, social needs, and reactions to physiological responses in various cultures produce different ways of defining and managing health and illness. It is important for those who provide women's health care to be aware of not only the cultural diversity, but also the limitations or constraints such diversity may present.

The unique population of this study makes the results difficult to generalize but still valuable. Some sources of bias in using a convenient sample are readily apparent, including "volunteerism." The FHCR was used for only 4 weeks of the study and a total of 14 emotinally related illnesses were reported. As with most studies, more questions are raised than answered. The findings from this study indicate that similar studies should be conducted with other populations

to further establish relationships between ideology and illness symptoms. Just how and in what ways belief systems that reinforce sexual
asymmetry influence women's health behavior are timely issues. The
results of this study indicate that women's heritage, including their
history through the progress of civilization, their current socialization, and the cultural context in which they live, influence their
behavior with respect to health and illness.

REFERENCES

Adams, R. N. (1970). *Crucifixion by power*. Austin: University of Texas Press.
Beals, R. L. (1952). Notes on acculturation. In S. Tax (Ed.), *Heritage of con-
quest*. Glencoe: The Free Press.
Beck, L., & Keddie, N. (1973). *Women in the Muslim world*. Cambridge: Har-
vard University Press.
De la Fuente, J. (1967). Ethnic relationships. In M. Nash (Ed.), *Handbook of
Middle American Indians: Social Anthropology* (Vol. 6). Austin: University
of Texas Press.
O'Kelley, C. G. (1980). *Women and men in society*. New York: van Nostrand.
Stevens, E. P. (1973). Marianismo: The other face of machismo. In A. Pescatello
(Ed.), *Female and male in Latin America*. Pittsburgh: University of Pittsburgh
Press.

PERCEPTIONS OF PROBLEMATIC BEHAVIOR BY SOUTHERN FEMALE BLACK FUNDAMENTALISTS AND MENTAL HEALTH PROFESSIONALS

**L. Marie Allen, RN, EdD, Phyllis B. Graves, RN, DSN,
and Elizabeth S. Woodward, RN, PhD**

Northwestern State University College of Nursing, Shreveport, Louisiana

Perceptions of problematic behavior by mental health professionals were found to be significantly different from those of a sample of Southern black female fundamentalists. Ten vignettes, each describing problematic behaviors, were used to elicit responses that were dichotomized as "mental illness/no mental illness," and "treatment/ no treatment." Among the fundamentalists, most "no mental illness" responses were related to religious belief. Other responses labeled behaviors as immoral, criminal, or psychic. Types of management recommended by black subjects often included prayer and religious counseling. These findings support the notion that transcultural nursing studies should pay attention to those religious beliefs that may underlie what is perceived as "normal" or "abnormal."

PURPOSE

The purpose of this study was to compare the perceptions of problematic behavior (Flaskerud, 1980) by mental health professionals with those of a sample of black female fundamentalists. The study was part of a national effort by Flaskerud to enlist nurse researchers in a broad sampling of lay minority groups (groups that can be distinguished by a shared set of cultural or religious norms) and mental health professionals such as nurses, physicians, and social workers.

CONCEPTS

The conceptual framework for the study consisted of the following:

This study was supported by a grant from the Council of University Research Administrators Institute, Northwestern State University of Louisiana.

Dominant culture: A collectivity of socially transmitted beliefs, patterns of behavior, institutions, and all other products of human work and thought characteristic of the members of a nation.

Minority subculture: A cultural subgroup, coexistent with a dominant culture but differentiated from it by status, ethnic background, religion, politics, residence, or other factors that unify the group and act on each member in a collective sense.

Religious belief system: A body of tenets, accepted on faith or trust, that are derived from shared perceptions of the powers and actions of a supernatural Being in relationships with humans.

PROBLEM DESCRIPTION

In spite of the changes that have moved the treatment of many of the mentally ill to the community and established the concept of "therapeutic community" within what were once custodial institutions, mental health-psychiatric nursing continues to be dominated by psychopathologically oriented traditions of clinical psychiatry (Osborne, 1973) that tend to standardize all forms of mental illness, behaviors that are regarded as symptoms of such illness, and the management of these behaviors. Flaskerud (1980) stated that psychiatric nursing, as it is now practiced and taught, continues to rely heavily on psychiatric medicine for labeling problematic behavior, and on psychiatric therapies for its management. This reliance has continued, although there is indication from transcultural studies

> . . . that neither the explanations for problematic behavior nor its management are standardized. Some minority groups (socioeconomic, religious, and ethnic) do not share psychiatry's explanations of which behaviors are normal and which abnormal, nor do they advocate the same types of management. . . . (Flaskerud, 1980, p. 4).

The relationship between culture and mental illness has been studied more frequently from an epidemiological perspective than from a perspective of cultural difference and perception of mental illness. Epidemiological studies can do much to pinpoint possible factors that are associated with the occurrence of mental illness, but they also tend to perpetuate the myth that certain minority groups, particularly blacks, have more mental illness than do whites (Thomas & Sellen, 1972).

Studies of interrelationships of cultural differences, illness perception, and health and healing practices have become more numerous in recent years (e.g., Fabrega, 1972; Kay, 1972; Scott, 1974; Stern, 1981). However few of the studies available in recent literature have dealt specifically with beliefs and practices regarding mental health among American subcultures.

Abel and Metraux (1974) discussed the difficulties encountered in dealing with psychopathologies in different cultural contexts, attitudes toward treatment, and problems in communication in therapy. Their studies have been chiefly concerned with some of the Caribbean groups that are forming communities within the United States. The studies of Giordano (1973) and Giordano and Levine (1975) dealt with interrelations between ethnicity and mental health and the problems created by these relationships; their studies have been made among white ethnic groups in the United States. The studies of these investigators have been oriented toward problems of medical anthropology and psychiatry, and are principally descriptive in nature. None has made use of vignettes to elicit broad concepts of mental health and illness among different cultural and/or ethnic groups (Flaskerud, 1979). In none of the studies that dealt with mental health and psychopathologies (Abel & Metraux, 1974; Giordano, 1973; Giordano & Levine, 1975), is there indication that the researchers recognized the emotional resistance, produced by their own culture and advanced education, that can impair the ability of professionals to apply any standards except their own to the perception of problematic behavior and its management (Murphy, 1972; Rawnsley, 1972).

The study of Karno and Edgerton (1969) was perhaps one of the earliest in which vignettes were used to elicit perceptions of mental illness in a minority group. The study was made in two subcommunities of Los Angeles: one Mexican-American, the other an Anglo community. Although the Mexican-Americans, in comparison to the Anglos, were "underrepresented" (p. 233) as psychiatric patients in local treatment centers, the researchers concluded that they did not ". . . perceive and define mental illness in significantly different ways than . . . Anglos" (p. 237). However, there were differences in cultural perceptions and customs of managing what was designated by the researchers as "mental illness."

Murray's study of perceptions of problematic behavior by three different groups (1978) was perhaps the first to compare minority group perceptions with those of mental health professionals and a lay nonminority group. Murray characterized the mental health professionals and lay nonminority respondents as representative of the dominant American culture, and hypothesized that there would be a significant difference between cultural groups in their interpretations and labeling of problematic behaviors described by vignettes in a structured interview. Murray's findings supported her hypothesis;

for example, behaviors labeled by the mental health professionals and lay nonminority subjects as "mental illness," requiring psychiatric management, were labeled by minority group subjects as (variously) lazy, mean, immoral, criminal, and psychic. Minority subjects tended to recommend punishment (mostly by one's own group) or tolerance of the behaviors.

Using an ethnoscientific approach, Bush, Ultom, and Osborne (1975) studied the meaning of mental health as conceptualized by male and female residents of a central city area and by male and female mental health professionals. They found that many activities considered "illegal" by society and labeled "sociopathic" by psychiatrists, were considered "mentally healthy" by some of their lay respondents, particularly the males. Their findings raised the question of sex differences in conceptualizing "mental health," and whether ethnic origin or socioeconomic grouping help to determine concepts and experiences associated with "mental health" (p. 137).

The implication of the findings of these studies is that there are possible cultural and sexual variations in defining mental health and labeling mental illness, and that what is viewed as abnormal behavior by one culture may be considered normal in another.

The major thrust in transcultural nursing, since its introduction as a subdiscipline in 1965 (Leininger, 1978), has been to promote knowledge about cultural differences and to apply this knowledge in nursing care situations. Most nurses view transcultural nursing from the perspective of health care values and practices in a subculture, as these may vary from those of the dominant culture (Leininger, 1976). A more comprehensive view would encompass a deeper understanding of those features of a cultural social structure that may influence perceptions of "normal" and "abnormal."

One feature of the social structure of minority subcultures that can be vitally important to such perceptions is religion. Religious ideology provides values that can determine health care norms and practices and influence the way in which group members perceive and label behaviors. Where these perceptions differ from those of mental health professionals, it is important that such differences be discovered and made known.

RELIGION AND THE BLACK SUBCULTURE

Religion has traditionally played an important role in the lives of black Americans (Pinkney, 1975). In black communities, the church has most often been the one institution blacks could call their own; it offered them opportunities for self-expression, leadership, and recognition. The church was the primary source of support in gaining pride through self-help, was important in maintaining group unity, and fostered self-respect (Hudson, 1965, p. 225). The black church has served as agency for both social control and socialization (Scanzoni, 1971). Religion and church life formed the foundation of a value system that made possible the accommodation of blacks to their status in the white man's society, particularly in the South (Frazier, 1971). The core of this value system, said Frazier, was "quiescence and faithful endurance" (p. 134) with the implication of a reward in Heaven.

There are perhaps 30 black Christian denominations, but seven of eight black church members is a Baptist or a Methodist. The most numerous are Baptists, with more than 9 million members. Black Baptists are generally thought to be more fundamentalist in their beliefs than are Methodists (Pinkney, 1975).

Although they are being welcomed into white churches in some areas of the South, most blacks continue to worship in "black" churches. Perhaps this is due to what Smith sees as a basic difference in white and black religion: white religion, he stated, is a cultural religion of "the flag, motherhood, and apple pie"; black religion is one of liberation and freedom (1976, p. 13).

Fundamentalism

A fundamentalist is perceived by most Americans as one who believes in the literal truth of the Bible. Rosten defined a fundamentalist as "one who believes in the infallibility of the Bible as inspired by God, and that it should be accepted literally" (1975, p. 640). Herman, in his study of the intellectual development of fundamentalism, found this to be the first of five tenets of fundamentalism; the others were Christ's virgin birth, His substitionary atonement for the sins of mankind, His resurrection in the flesh, and His supernatural miracles. Sandeen traces the roots of fundamentalism to the Niagara Creed of 1878; the Creed had 14 points, the first of which was that all scripture is given by inspiration of God, and this divine inspiration extends fully and equally to every word of the Bible (1970, p. 273).

Hudson affirmed that a fundamentalist is generally perceived in this manner, and that "Southern Protestants are universally said to be fundamentalists" (1972, p. 122). Hudson went on to point out the basic flaw in this definition; that is, that many so-called fundamentalists may be illiterate, and if so, it would be astonishing to require literal acceptance of the Bible as a "prerequisite for access to their system of belief" (p. 122). What then, he asked, are the essential tenets of a fundamentalist belief system?

It was Hudson's work in constructing this belief system from his study of white fundamentalists that revealed the fact that black fundamentalism has never been studied. It was therefore necessary for the investigators in the present study, following the methods of Hudson and using his concepts, to construct a belief system by questioning a sample of female members of the same church from which the study sample was drawn.

Belief System of Southern Black Fundamentalists

The belief system of the black fundamentalists in the present study consists chiefly of how they perceive God, the mind, Satan (or the devil), and how these relate to the lives and souls of human beings. According to our data the beliefs of southern black fundamentalists can be summarized in the following ways:

God is perceived as omnipotent and omniscient; He has a hand in everything and can cause events to happen. God is in the mind as conscience or feeling, but He also communicates externally through signs and warnings that must be carefully and thoughtfully interpreted. A southern black fundamentalist female may say, "Why me, Lord?", but still accepts what is perceived as God's will; it is not wise for humans to try to understand all God's mysteries.

Satan, or the devil, is the embodiment of evil and temptations that draw people away from the Hand of God. Satan can be in the mind of a person or he can communicate with a person from external sources.

The Mind is the seat of the Soul, and it is God's greatest gift to an individual. The mind allows the person to make decisions about his life and his relationship with God. The most important qualities of the mind are faith and will; faith makes it possible for a person to have confidence in ultimately good outcomes, will gives the person the power to resist the wiles of Satan. Newborn babies have no mind in the sense of conscience or feeling, but they have the capacity to develop this as they mature. It is during this period when they are maturing that the struggle between God and Satan for control of the mind is most intense; it is then that they must be saved from Satan and become children of God. This is *Salvation.*

Salvation cannot happen until a person is mature enough in mind to perceive the will of God. Salvation can take place anywhere, but it is more liberating for the mind if it takes place in church; there are others present who are helping, through their prayers, to liberate a mind from the devil. Salvation is a significant social and ideological event; once a person has been saved he is more worthy to be a part of the community, and he is ready to obey God and look to Him for guidance. A person is always saved through Jesus.

Blessings are good things that happen to people; they are not evenly distributed, but can happen to bad people as well as good people. Those events that cannot be explained are part of the mysteries in the way God works in the lives of humans. It is God who fixes the time and circumstances of one's death, and it is sinful to do anything to try to alter His will in this (for example, by attempting suicide).

The Bible is God's Word, and it is literal truth to those who have achieved Salvation. Being saved helps one to interpret and understand the Word of God, with help from those who have studied the Word.

STUDY QUESTIONS AND HYPOTHESES

Questions

The general questions this study asked were: What are the differences between groups in the name or label each applies to a set of behaviors? What are the differences between groups in suggested management of each set of behaviors?

Hypotheses

It was hypothesized that:

1. There will be a significant difference between members of a black fundamentalist minority group and mental health professionals in the number of behaviors labeled "mental illness."
2. There will be a significant difference between members of a black fundamentalist minority group and mental health professionals in the frequency with which psychiatric management of the behaviors is recommended.

INSTRUMENT

The data collection instrument was an interview schedule developed by Flaskerud (1980) to measure subjects' views of problematic behavior and its management and to provide demographic data. The 10 vignettes in the instrument, which are included in the Appendix at the end of this paper, present short, compact descriptions of problematic behavior.

Content of the vignettes was based on review of the literature and records of individuals who were members of a minority who had been hospitalized for mental illness (Flaskerud, 1979). Behaviors described in the vignettes were selected to be representative of behaviors specific to minority cultures and typical of mental illness in the majority culture. Validity of the vignettes was established by a panel of experts and pretesting.

After the interviewer reads each vignette, the subject is asked the following questions. First, "What do you think of this man's (woman's) behavior?" Second, "Do you think anything ought to be done about this matter?" If the subject responds affirmatively to question two, a third question, "What do you think ought to be done?" is asked. Responses yield both qualitative and quantitative data. To obtain quantitative data, responses to question one are dichotomized and categorized as mental illness or no mental illness and responses to question three are dichotomized and categorized as psychiatric treatment or no psychiatric treatment.

DATA COLLECTION

Data from all subjects were collected by personal interview. A sample of convenience was used both for the black fundamentalist group and for the mental health professional group.

A convenience sample of mental health professionals was drawn from a medical center, a neuro-psychiatric hospital, a group practice of psychiatrists and clinical social workers, and students enrolled in a graduate program in mental health-psychiatric nursing leading to the Master of Science in Nursing degree. All who were asked to participate agreed to do so and no one available at the time of data collection was excluded.

Random sampling is indicated as the method of choice in selection of subjects. In spite of inherent problems regarding generalizability when a nonprobability sample is used and the limitations due to population size in the given locale, the investigators chose to employ convenience sampling with all its limitations on the study findings.

SUBJECTS

Two groups of respondents, 20 black female fundamentalists and 20 mental health professionals, comprised the sample. With the exception of one mental health professional, subjects were born and reared in the United States. All black female fundamentalists were members of Baptist congregations and attended services regularly. Although all mental health professionals identified themselves as having a religion, five responded that they did not attend church or synagogue. Among mental health professionals, 16 were Protestant, including 6 Baptists; two were Catholic and two were Jewish. Age, sex, race, and education of subjects in the two groups is given in Table 1. Black female fundamentalists tended to be older and less well educated than mental health professionals. Because of selection criteria (not applied to mental health professionals) all in the fundamentalist group were women and were black.

Occupations among the fundamentalists were varied and included blue-collar, white-collar, and professional positions. Five of the women in this group were not employed; one was a student, two were housewives, and two were retired.

Mental health professionals included one psychologist, one social worker, one counselor, and 17 psychiatric nurses. Places of employment were psychiatric services in general hospitals, a neuropsychi-

Table 1. Age, Sex, Race, and Education of Subjects

	Black female fundamentalists	Mental health professionals
Age		
Range	24–79	24–61
Mean	46	36
Sex		
Female	20	15
Male	0	5
Race		
Black	20	2
White	0	18
Education		
Less than high school	7	0
Some college or high school	8	5
College or advanced degree	5	15

atric hospital, a mental health center, and private practice. The length of time they had been in their work situations ranged from 3 weeks to 19 years with a mean of 5 years.

DATA ANALYSIS

The data were analyzed in two ways. The primary analysis dealt with the stated hypotheses of difference between the two groups in (1) how the behavior should be labeled and (2) how the behavior should be treated. Secondary to this was an analysis of the relationship between the demographic variables and the labeling and treatment of the described behavior.

The sample size and the data format suggested use of the nonparametric statistic chi-square. The use of a convenience sample supports this choice but limits the internal and external validity of the conclusions.

To analyze the data, chi-square contingency tables were employed. Since some expected cell frequencies were less than five, Yates' correction for continuity was applied to all chi-square values (Ferguson, 1981).

For each vignette two analyses were conducted. The first was a 2 X 2 table representing a fundamentalist/mental health professional by illness/no illness analysis. The second analysis was fundamentalist/mental health professional by treatment/no treatment contingency. As Table 2 reveals, all analyses, with the exception of one, were significant at the .05 level.

Table 2. Chi Square Values for All Vignettes

Vignette	Illness/no illness	Treatment/no treatment
1	20.91	23.44
2	4.90	4.90
3	14.73	14.73
4	9.18	14.40
5	15.36	15.36
6	7.66	10.81
7	9.18	7.66
8	3.65	4.90
9	16.41	18.57
10	20.91	14.73

FINDINGS

The results of the analysis concerning perception of behavior and the need for treatment are displayed in Table 2. All probabilities for these values are significant ($df = 1$) at the .05 level except for vignette eight responses to the question concerning mental illness/no mental illness.

On the nine vignettes of significance, the mental health professionals were more likely to classify the behavior as indicative of mental illness than the fundamentalist minority group. On the tenth vignette, the consensus of both groups was mental illness. These findings support acceptance of hypothesis one.

Responses from the mental health professionals to the question of treatment/no treatment for each of the persons described in the vignettes was significantly different from those of the black fundamentalist minority group. These findings support acceptance of hypothesis two.

PERCEPTIONS OF BEHAVIOR

Responses to the question "What do you think of this man's (woman's) behavior?" which followed each of the 10 vignettes were classified as "mental illness" or "no mental illness." A majority (55%) of the responses of the fundamentalists fell in the category "no mental illness." The most frequently occurring "no mental illness" responses related to religion. Typical answers were: "It's God's plan," "Full of sin," "Is talking to God," and "The devil is in him." This type of statement accounted for 22% of the "no mental illness" responses. Examples of other kinds of answers are: immoral behavior, "She's using her beauty the wrong way;" psychic, "Special intuition;" medical problem, "It may be due to a dietary problem;" and criminal, "It's wrong."

Fundamentalist subjects' responses among those included in the category mental illness were: "Psychological problem," "Nutty," "Mental trouble," "Crazy," and "Nervous." Only rarely did subjects in this group use terms such as depression or schizophrenic.

The mental health professionals tended to view the behavior described in each vignette as psychotic (35%), mentally sick (35%), or emotionally disturbed (30%). The mental health professionals avoided the use of diagnostic terms in 18 (90%) of the cases. Responses included such broad terms as psychotic, mentally ill, sick, and crazy, among others.

PERCEPTIONS OF MANAGEMENT

Subjects were asked whether anything should be done about the behavior described in each vignette and if the response was yes, what ought to be done. Black female fundamentalists indicated that nonpsychiatric treatment was most frequently (46%) their choice of behavior management. Psychiatric treatment was suggested 41% of the time. Thirteen percent of the responses indicated no management was needed.

Among the nonpsychiatric managements, individual and/or family coping without outside assistance was often suggested. Examples were: "Be more involved," "Talk with his wife," "Get job training," "Ignore it," and "Parents should talk with her." Support from caring persons was also frequently suggested; "Needs love, a caring person," "Needs someone to trust," and "A husband or friend to talk with her."

Other kinds of nonpsychiatric management suggested by the fundamentalist group included prayer, religious counseling, incarceration, and medical treatment. Generally, when the behavior described in a vignette posed no threat, subjects would tend to recommend either no management or nonpunitive management.

When psychiatric treatment was the management suggested by the fundamentalist group, most often a mental health professional was identified; for example "See a psychiatrist." Psychiatrists, psychologists, and social workers were the professionals named. It is interesting to note that nurses were not mentioned by subjects in this group. Neither did the subjects recommend specific therapies such as medication.

As in the response of the members of the fundamentalist group, the mental health professionals did not mention the psychiatric nurse as an appropriate treatment resource. This was true in spite of the fact that 17 (85%) of the subjects were nurses and 14 (70%) were currently employed in an acute care psychiatric hospital.

The impact of the trend toward community based treatment or management of even the psychotic individual was reflected in the choice of treatment. Responses of the fundamentalist group indicated hospitalization as the treatment of choice only 13% of the time. A majority either specified no treatment setting (81%) or an outpatient setting (33%). Treatment in an outpatient setting was selected by the mental health professionals 40% of the time and hospitalization was recommended in only 15% of the cases. Forty-five percent of the responses made no distinction between outpatient and inpatient approaches to the care believed to be needed.

RESEARCH IMPLICATIONS

Because this study was of black females only, there remain the questions of possible sex difference in perceptions of mental illness, and whether or not the belief system of the black females would be affirmed in a similar study of black males. Further, since there have been no prior studies of black fundamentalist belief systems, this feature of the social structure of black subcultures should be studied. Knowledge of differences in belief systems among other denominations of black Christians and in other regions of the United States would add needed depth to our scant knowledge of values systems that may underlie health care norms and practices, as well as perceptions of what is normal and what is abnormal.

The frequency with which respondents identified outpatient treatment or treatment without specifying environment rather than institutionalized treatment was a serendipitous finding of the study. The study questions focused on the decisions regarding a mental illness versus nonmental illness and treatment versus nontreatment and resulted in dichotomous data. The question of location and type of treatment are more appropriately represented as continua. The location of treatment could vary from institutionalization with no community based activity and total structure of environment to a community agency offering psychological support on demand with a significant self-care component. The type of treatment would include at one extreme individual therapy and at the other family or group therapy. With the existing variation in both the variables of location and treatment mode, and the fervor with which each is supported by its adherents, a study of these variables could provide an interesting and informative insight to both the public and professional perception of the relationship between problematic behavior and the course and site of treatment. The data obtained in this study clearly indicate the existence of opinions on the two questions.

SUMMARY

The findings of this study are consistent with those of Murray (1978), in which the vignettes were used to elicit differences between mental health professionals and minority groups in their perceptions of problematic behavior and its management. Minorities in both studies tended to have a broader perspective of problematic behavior and its related treatment than did mental health professionals.

Since the black females in this study may be said to perceive the mind as God's most important gift to an individual, and the mind as the seat of the soul, it seems reasonable to conclude that, rather than perceiving aberrant behavior as "mental illness" requiring medical treatment, it is more natural that they perceive such behavior as phenomena that might be corrected or cured through recourse to the powers of God.

Incorporation of transcultural health care values and practices may be inadequate unless the nurse seeks to understand the belief system underlying those values and practices. This more basic understanding leads to acceptance of clients on their own terms and can lead to identification of similarities that transcend the more obvious cultural classifications.

The repeated references by the fundamentalist group to the need for emotional support in the care of people with problematic behavior lend strength to the idea that it is necessary for nurses to include families and significant others among the resources available to clients. It is interesting that these responses were not among those of the mental health professionals.

Neither subjects in the fundamentalist minority group nor subjects in the mental health professional group identified psychiatric nurses as a resource for management of problematic behavior. Current developments in the practice role of the mental health-psychiatric nurse include joint practice agreements with psychiatrists and clinical psychologists, independent practice, and changes in employee classification within health care agencies allowing advanced practice. Increased numbers of master's prepared mental health-psychiatric nurses have made these changes possible. It will be interesting to note in the future whether these changes will result in a change in the perception of nurses as a source of treatment.

REFERENCES

Abel, T., & Metraux, R. (1974). *Culture and psychotherapy.* New Haven: College and University Press.

Bush, M. T., Ultom, J. A., & Osborne, O. H. (1975). The meaning of mental health: A report of two ethnoscientific studies. *Nursing Research, 24,* 130–138.

Fabrega, H., Jr. (1972). Medical anthropology. In B. Siegel (Ed.), *Biennial review of anthropology,* Vol. 7. Stanford: Stanford University Press.

Flaskerud, J. H. (1979). Use of vignettes to elicit broad concepts. *Nursing Research, 28,* 210–212.

Flaskerud, J. H. (1980). A tool for comparing the perceptions of problematic behavior by psychiatric professionals and minority groups. *Nursing Research, 29,* 4–9.

Ferguson, G. A. (1981). *Statistical analysis in psychology and education* (5th ed.) (p. 214). New York: McGraw-Hill.

Frazier, E. F. (1971). The Negro church and assimilation. In H. M. Nelsen, R. L. Yokley, and A. F. Nelsen (Eds.), *The black church in America* (pp. 131–140). New York: Basic.

Giordano, J. (1973). *Ethnicity and mental health: Research and recommendations.* New York: The Institute on Pluralism and Group Identity.

Giordano, J., & Levine, M. (1975). *Mental health and middle America: A group identity approach.* New York: The Institute on Pluralism and Group Identity.

Herman, D. E. (1980). *Flooding the kingdom: The intellectual development of fundamentalism, 1930-1941.* Unpublished doctoral dissertation, Ohio University Athens.

Hudson, C. (1972). The structure of a fundamentalist Christian belief system. In S. S. Hill, Jr., E. T. Thompson, A. F. Scott, C. Hudson, and E. S. Gaustad (Eds.), *Religion and the solid South* (pp. 122–142), Nashville: Abingdon.

Hudson, W. S. (1965). *Religion in America* (p. 225). New York: Scribner.

Karno, M., & Edgerton, R. B. (1969). Perception of mental illness in a Mexican-American community. *Archives of General Psychiatry, 20,* 233–238.

Kay, M. A. (1972). *Health and illness in the barrio: Women's point of view.* Unpublished doctoral dissertation, University of Arizona, Tucson.

Leininger, M. M. (1976). *Transcultural health care: Issues and conditions.* Philadelphia: Davis.

Leininger, M. M. (1978). *Transcultural nursing: Concepts, theories, and practices.* New York: Wiley.

Murphy, H. B. M. (1972). Current trends in transcultural psychiatry. *Proceedings of The Royal Society of Medicine, 66,* 711–717.

Murray, J. H. (1978). *Perceptions of problematic behavior by Appalachians, mental health professionals, and lay non-Appalachians.* Unpublished doctoral dissertation, The University of Illinois at the Medical Center, Chicago.

Osborne, O. H. (1973). Anthropological issues in mental health nursing. In M. M. Leininger (Ed.), *Contemporary issues in mental health nursing* (pp. 39–61). Boston: Little Brown.

Pinkney, A. (1975). *Black Americans* (2nd ed.). Englewood Cliffs, NJ: Prentice Hall.

Rownsley, K. (1972). Discussion. *Proceedings of the Royal Society of Medicine, 66,* 718.

Rosten, L. (Ed.) (1975). *Religions of America: Ferment and faith in an age of crisis.* New York: Simon & Schuster.

Sandeen, E. R. (1970). *The roots of fundamentalism: British and American millenarianism, 1800-1930.* Chicago: University of Chicago Press.

Scanzoni, J. H. (1971). *The black family in modern society.* Boston: Allyn & Bacon.

Scott, C. S. (1974). Health and healing practices among five ethnic groups in Miami, Florida. *Public Health Reports, 89,* 524–532.

Smith, J. A. (1976). The role of the black clergy as allied health professionals in working with black patients. In D. Luckraft (Ed.), *Black awareness.* New York: American Journal of Nursing.

Stern, P. N. (1981). Resolving problems of health care teaching: The Filipino child-bearing family. *Image XIII*, pp. 47–50.

Thomas, A., & Sellen, S. (1972). *Racism and psychiatry.* New York: Brunner-Mazel.

APPENDIX: VIGNETTES USED
IN THE SURVEY INSTRUMENT

1. The first person is a 42-year-old woman who was married and and has five children. Several years ago her husband left her and she does not know where he is. Since that time she has become very religious and spends a lot of time each week at church services and prayer meetings. She believes that she has special powers from God. She claims that on many occasions she has seen Jesus surrounded by his angels. She gets very excited and emotional on these occasions. She cries, moans, throws herself on the floor and talks loudly to Jesus and his angels. She says that she has healed other people because of her faith. Her older children feel that she spends too much time on these activities and that she neglects the younger ones.

2. This next person is a 40-year-old man who is married. He is a very suspicious person. Sometimes he thinks that people he sees on the street are talking about him or following him around. A couple of times now, he has beaten up men who did not even know him because he thought that they were plotting against him. The other night he began to curse his wife terribly; then he hit her and threatened to kill her because, he said, she was working against him too just like everyone else.

3. This is a 24-year-old woman who is unmarried. She looks younger than 24 years—about 17 or 18 and she speaks in a very soft, young voice. She has had some hard times in her life. Although she is not married, she has two children by different fathers. Right now she lives alone with the children but she has a hard time taking care of them and handling them. She has been arrested twice for soliciting and once for causing a disturbance on the street. Each time she has been in jail she has become very upset and hysterical—crying loudly, throwing herself on the floor, and refusing to eat. When she is released, she tries hard to be a good mother but her attempts at it do not last very long and soon she is in trouble again.

4. This is a 42-year-old man who is divorced. His ex-wife and two children live here in (city) but he has not seen them in years. He thinks he has special mental powers and that he receives messages through electrical waves that other people cannot hear. Most of these messages are about danger to the United States from foreign, com-

munist countries. He tries very hard to get in touch with the President of the United States and the governor to warn them of nuclear attacks. The messages he hears tell him that the United States is going to be bombed and he tries to warn the government of these attacks. People in government ignore him and do not answer his letters or phone calls.

5. This individual is a 35-year-old woman who is married. She has experienced episodes for the last several years in which she can see figures of spirits standing around her and she can also sometimes hear voices mumbling to her. No one else can see or hear these things. During these experiences, she talks in a strange, low-pitched tone of voice and reveals messages from the spirits. These episodes may last anywhere from a few hours to a week. Between episodes, she carries on her regular activities but is not very outgoing.

6. This is a woman who is 30 years old, married, and has three children. Every day she cries and weeps for hours on end and does not take care of her children. She claims that all kinds of people are accusing her of trying to hurt them. She feels that her thoughts and deeds may have harmed thousands of people. She thinks and talks about killing herself. She sits for hours without moving. She does not take a bath, wash, comb her hair, or change her clothes.

7. This is a man who is 30 years old, married, and has four children. He is a very quiet man; he does not talk much and he does not trust or like strangers or bosses. He works in a factory but does not have much hope of getting ahead in life. Every night after work he drinks in a bar, sometimes coming home late at night. Sometimes he and his wife argue loudly about his drinking and on occasion during these arguments he hits her. Once when he was very angry with her, he bruised her face badly, broke windows in his apartment, and threw furniture into the street.

8. This is an 18-year-old girl who is in high school. She has always been a moody girl and has never gotten along well with people. A few months ago she began to cry all the time and act afraid of everyday things. She has stopped going to school and stays at home. She screams at her parents, and a lot of the time what she says does not make any sense to them. She has talked about hearing voices talk to her and thinks she is really somebody other than herself.

9. This is a 45-year-old man who is married and has three children. Although when he was younger he was full of life and a hard worker, now he is moody, stays at home a lot, and does not talk much. He is presently unemployed and complains of trouble with his nerves. He says he has pain in his back and legs and has been to many doctors who have not been able to find much wrong with him but they do

give him nerve medicine. His last job as a laborer on a truck dock, was, he says, too hard on his nerves. Now he sits at home most of the time, does not talk much, and lets his wife do things for him.

10. This is a man, aged 27, who is not married. Every now and then he sees the figure of his mother, who died a few years ago, standing before him. He then talks to her and she replies to him. People who are with him when he talks to his mother do not see or hear her. He is described by his friends as a rather excitable but friendly person.

CULTURALLY INDUCED STRESS DURING CHILDBEARING:
THE PILIPINO–AMERICAN EXPERIENCE

Phyllis Noerager Stern, DNS, RN, FAAN
Dalhousie University School of Nursing, Halifax, Nova Scotia

Virginia Peterson Tilden, RN, DNS
Oregon Health Science University, Portland, Oregon

Eleanor Krassen Maxwell, PhD
Kern County Economic Opportunities Corporation, Bakersfield, California

Pregnancy and childbearing have been rated as two of the most stressful events in any woman's life. In a group of Pilipino immigrants, additional stress was found to exist when their cultural values regarding self-care during pregnancy differed from those of their western health care givers. A sensitive attitude of the nurse toward custom approach and language was found to reduce stress felt by the childbearing Pilipino immigrant.

In this paper we discuss culturally induced stress associated with childbearing as identified in the findings of a field study of Pilipino-American families and their interactions with Western American

Tagalog, the national language of the Philippines, has no "F" sound; therefore, the spelling Pilipino and Pilipina used in this paper represents a more culturally sensitive report than the more familiar American version of Filipino or Filipina.

This study was supported in part by Faculty Development Grant #2-405231-09501, University of California, and by Biomedical Research Support Grant RR050604 from the Biomedical Research Support Branch, Division of Research Facilities and Resources, National Institutes of Health.

The authors wish to thank the administration and staff of the seven San Francisco Bay Area health care facilities who participated in this study: San Francisco General, Oakland Naval Regional Medical Center, South of Market Clinic, University of California, San Francisco Ambulatory Care Facility, Moffitt Hospital, and St. Luke's Hospital, San Francisco. Special thanks is due to Nellie Jocson, Director of Nursing Education, St. Luke's Hospital, and to the Pilipino Nurses of St. Luke's. We also wish to thank the Pilipino families who gave of their time so we might become better informed.

This paper has been substantially rewritten since it was first published in 1980 in *Issues in Health Care of Women, 2*(3–4).

Copyright © 1985 by Hemisphere Publishing Corporation

health professionals. Our data suggest that cultural differences between Western American health professionals create stressful variables during childbearing. Additionally, Western health providers'
ignorance of Pilipino cultural beliefs and folkways compound the
stressors. Perinatal research of the last several decades amply documents the disruptive role of stress in pregnancy outcome (McDonald,
1968), though no study has specifically explored culturally induced
perinatal stress.

Initially, we review research concerning the role of stress in childbearing. We then compare documented Pilipino childbirth experiences in the Philippine Islands with childbirth experiences following
immigration. Finally, we present our findings from 161 interviews
and 400 hours of observation. These findings indicate an increase in
psychological stress for women of Pilipino origin in Western American health care settings. Communication breakdown, and mutual
ignorance of health care beliefs, we found, interfere with psychological well-being during pregnancy and consequently with the learning
process when new health concepts are taught. Suggested interven-
tions are included.

CONCEPTUALIZATIONS AND RELEVANT LITERATURE

Social Process

Anthropological literature reveal a universal tendency for the creation of ceremonial rite around every important life event. Pregnancy
and childbearing, like death and dying, are especially imbued with
ritual. Deutsch (1945) writes that pregnant women of all cultures
and all eras experience fear of the evil spirits, or *vahina-hai,* in what
seems a universal and timeless anxiety inherent in the procreative
process. In response, pregnant women seek security measures and
court benevolent gods with ritualized behavior, whether anointing
their abdomens with herbal oils in an African village or practicing
daily yoga in California.

Protective rituals pass from model to protegé in the form of formal teaching, such as childbirth classes; informal teaching, as in
observation; and in folktales. Regardless of the locale, major life
events lead to the generation and passing on of exact ritual. In her
work on modeling in nonindustrial societies, Maxwell (1979) noted
that important life-cycle events dramatized by ritual provided excellent opportunities for older persons to teach their values to their
protegés. In addition to preparing novices for the experiences they

were about to undergo, elders served as models that young people could simulate since the elders had more or less successfully completed the experience that the novice was just beginning.

Modeling appears to be an especially important social process during pregnancy. Rubin (1967) describes the importance of peers as behavioral role models and referents as the novice assumes the maternal role. Female peers are selected and rejected on the basis of their suitability as models. Modeling is most evident in mother-daughter relationships. Women's pregnancies rekindle important issues in the relationship between a daughter and her mother surrogate (Ballou, 1978; Benedek, 1956). A need to reconcile conflict and renegotiate dependency lines predominates, regardless of whether or not the mother is physically present or even alive. The internalized mother, her caveats and behavioral prescriptions, must be entertained. Bibring (1961) suggests that a reworking of the mother-daughter relationship constitutes a development issue of pregnancy, the optimal outcome of which elevates the daughter to a new position of peer status with the mother, and the transfer of mother's libidinal energies to daughter to new grandchild. The quality of the original mother-daughter relationship helps to shape the character and quality of the new mother-infant relationship.

Psychological Process

Bibring (1959), Bibring, Dwyer, Huntington, and Valenstein (1961), Caplan (1961), and Shereshefsky and Yarrow (1973) suggest that pregnancy precipitates major id-ego disequilibria resulting in temporary ego function weakness and a triggering of unconscious psychological conflicts. These and other theorists (Cohen, 1979; Rubin, 1976) posit the necessity for pregnant women to master the following specific developmental tasks during pregnancy: 1) incorporation of the intruding fetus; 2) increasing emotional affiliation with the fetus; 3) relating to the fetus as a separate object after quickening, nesting behavior, and emotional preparation for delivery; and 4) letting go of the fetus at birth and binding in with the neonate through the process of bonding and attachment.

Thus, social and psychological process attending childbearing serve important functions in ensuring safe passage, realigning relationships and preparing for transition to the maternal role. Such processes are universal phenomena of childbearing. When cultural prescriptions for behavior during childbearing are congruent with women's internalized prescriptions provided by female ancestry, harmonious forces accompany her developmental progression throughout the childbearing year. If current cultural prescriptions conflict with those internalized earlier from a prior culture, as in the case of transplanted Pilipinos, cultural dichotomy results, predisposing such women to heightened anxiety and developmental mastery failure.

Role of Stress in Pregnancy Outcome

Research indicates that women stressed during their pregnancies have higher rates of obstetrical pathology (Gorsuch & Key, 1974; Norbeck & Tilden, 1983; Nuckolls, Cassell, & Kaplin, 1972; Uddenberg & Fagerstrom, 1976) and longer and more difficult labors and deliveries (Crawford, 1968; Lederman, Lederman, Work, & McCann, 1978). Stress also plays a subtle role in shaping a woman's mental image of her fetus and later in the kind of relationship she develops with her newborn (Cranley, 1981; Cohen, 1966). McDonald (1968) concludes that anxiety during pregnancy of sufficient intensity and duration results in adaptive coping failure. This failure becomes manifest in one or more of a myriad of pregnancy complications, the exact nature of which depends on the individual and her specific constitution and genetic predisposition.

Certain kinds of stress prove most disruptive to women during pregnancy. Helper, Cohen, Beiteman, and Eaton (1968) have identified four categories: 1) any adverse event that the woman perceives as having the potential to damage her fetus; 2) any defect or conflict in the woman's support system, particularly involving mother or mate; 3) the woman's perception that she is poorly prepared, inexperienced, or otherwise inadequate to assume the maternal role; 4) any maternal condition that the woman believes might be worsened by the pregnancy. These categories are useful in understanding stress experienced by women raised in disparate cultures receiving Western style prenatal care. Such cultural dichotomy leads to stress of this very nature.

Role of Social Support in Pregnancy Outcome

Social support has been identified as a major variable in adaptation to stressful life events. Research findings of the past decade document the significant role played by social support in moderating stress and preventing negative health consequences. As discussed above, theorists on the psychology of pregnancy have addressed the important role played by family and friends in the social construction of the pregnancy experience (Ballou, 1978; Rubin, 1967).

Other researchers documented statistically significant correlations between aspects of social support and rates of pregnancy complications. Nuckolls et al. (1972) measured life stress and psychosocial assets of 170 normal primiparas, correlating those variables with the rate of complications. In small subsamples, women low in assets (including but not limited to social support) had three times the rate of complications than women high in assets. In a separate study of similar design, Norbeck and Tilden (1983) found that in a sample of 117 normal primiparas and multiparas, women who scored high stress in the year prior to the pregnancy had a significantly higher rate of complications. Further, women who scored high in stress during the pregnancy and low in social support, scored significantly higher in each of the three types of complications: gestation complications, labor and delivery complications, and neonatal complications. Both of these studies indicate that social support not only facilitates women's subjective sense of well-being during pregnancy, but has an important influence on health outcomes.

Immigration and cultural dichotomy alter normal social support network structure. Social supportive behaviors may be highly valued by a culture, but the disruption of immigration can seriously weaken network ties. In general, needs of social support at any one time are determined jointly by properties of the situation and properties of the person (Norbeck, 1981). Cross culturally, women report increased need for social support during the maturational crisis of pregnancy. Asian cultures prescribe many highly visible supportive interpersonal behaviors. For example, when a person is hospitalized the expectation is that the extended family and many friends will be present frequently, even in the intensive care unit. This expectation differs from that of Westerners during hospitalization. The event of immigration may place a pregnant woman at risk for lower quality and quantity of social support than perceived needed by the woman.

Pilipino-American Women

About 38,000 Pilipino immigrants arrive in the United States each year (U.S. Bureau of the Census, 1978). Some 60,000 Pilipino-Americans reside in the San Francisco Bay Area alone. Although constituting a large minority group, they remain relatively invisible, while other Americans are generally ignorant of Pilipino customs. Despite the size of this ethnic minority, studies that deal with care for transplanted Pilipinos are markedly lacking. Kalish and Yuen (1973) discuss problems of aging Pilipinos in the United States. Other accounts of the Pilipino experience in America may be found in Lott (1976) and Hunt (1954). Shon (1972) and Duff and Arthur

(1973) separately explored the effect of transplantation on the mental health of Pilipinos. The Pilipino belief in nonaggressive behavior and their intense fear of shaming self and family are the subjects of both these works.

A literature search located only one study of Pilipino childbearing in the United States: Affonso's (1975) work on childbirth perceptions. Her study of 65 Pilipina women living in Hawaii revealed a retained core of folk beliefs as well as a generally positive attitude toward children and childbearing. The study we present here is unique in its focus on the interaction between health care professionals and Pilipina childbearing women in the United States.

METHODOLOGY

The present study employed traditional field research methods of participant observation and interviewing to gather data on the interactions of Pilipino-American childbearing families and Western health professionals. Data collected over a 12-month period in 1978 and 1979 consisted of 161 interviews and over 400 hours of observation. Subjects were 40 Pilipino-American pregnant or postpartal women, 10 husbands and 10 mothers of the women, 40 registered nurses, 35 licensed vocational nurses, 6 physicians, and 20 student nurses. All interviews and observation took place at San Francisco Bay Area health care facilities, consisting of three general hospitals and three out-patient clinics. Three nurse researchers familiar with maternity patients and maternity health care settings conducted all interviews. Data were coded and ordered according to predominate processes (Glaser & Strauss, 1967; Stern, 1980; Stern, Allen, & Moxley, 1982) in the social context of communicating health teaching between Western providers and Pilipino-American childbearing women.

FINDINGS AND DISCUSSION

This study revealed that Pilipina women reared with non-Western models of childbearing often respond with stress during pregnancy when receiving Western obstetrical care. Although we observed a wide variety of responses that reflect individuality and certain regional differences, we were able to record a number of generalities in the data.

Flawed communication stemming from cultural conflict in three general areas generates stress:

1. Customs, cultural beliefs, and cultural practices associated with childbearing;
2. Interpersonal style leading to differences in social approach between recipients and providers of health care;
3. Language barriers created by cadence and accent, and variety and the use of idioms by health care providers.

Customs

Pilipino beliefs associated with childbearing are influenced by Catholicism, provincial custom, and Spanish-American colonization. Philippine Island provinces, however, many of which are separated by water, are diverse, therefore spawning a wide variety of cultural beliefs and practices.[*] Pilipino immigrants to the United States reflect the same diversity in their new home.

Health care in the cities of the Philippines resembles our own, the result of postwar recovery programs and of colonization. Even in remote provinces, American medicine is held in high esteem as an ideal model. Thus, while technology is less advanced than that of the US, women are accustomed to having babies in the hospital, attended by trained personnel.[†] Obstetrical personnel, however, are always other women, trained in the Philippines where allowances are made for cultural beliefs and where interpersonal styles mesh.

In the United States, health professionals are generally ignorant of Pilipino customs. Although professionals observe behaviors that are normally culturally correct for the Pilipino, many of them interpret these behaviors as resistance to teaching, rather than adherence to cultural beliefs. We were told by a few Western caregivers that Pilipino-American patients are "sneaky," "lazy," and "deceptive." Although generally sympathetic to the cultural beliefs of their fellow immigrants, caregivers of Pilipino origin that we observed did not pass on information regarding these beliefs to Western providers unless specifically asked.

---

[*]Anthropological ethnographies provide an abundant source of information for the scholar interested in Pilipino childbearing beliefs. Good examples are Nydegger and Nydegger's (1966) description of Tarong or Jacano's (1969) ethnography of the Malitbog Barrio. This paper presents a few representative customs discovered in our fieldwork, but no attempt was made to cover the vast array of native customs, as this discussion focuses on immigrant Pilipinos. Affonso (1978) presents an excellent overview of Pilipino customs.

[†]Based on personal conversation with Girl Scout Leaders on educational tour through Silliman University, Philippines, June 11, 1979, at University of California, San Francisco.

Diet and Medication

Beliefs regarding eating behavior are particularly relevant. Pilipinos hold that the pregnant women should eat a nourishing ethnic diet, but should refrain from eating any extra foods in order to keep the baby small in preparation for an easier delivery. Pregnant Pilipino women, never having acquired a taste for it, generally avoid drinking milk. A Pilipino dietitian explained:

> In the Philippines, you can't get milk, it's expensive, and if you have any, you save it for children. When you get it, it's canned, and then you reconstitute it with coconut milk. Pilipinos don't have the proper enzymes in their digestive systems to handle milk the way whites do.

Acquired taste seems a matter of small concern in many diet sheets distributed routinely to maternity patients. The assumption seems to be that one or possibly two ethnic groups live within the total United States. In some cases, items that appear on diet sheets are actually defined as taboo by Pilipinos from remote provinces. In some regions, for example, dark skinned fruits and vegetables are believed to darken the fetus' skin.

In addition to these dietary prohibitions, Pilipinas may follow certain ritual dietary inclusions. A common one in the Philippines involves the purchase of baby chicks during the first trimester of pregnancy. Raised during the gestational period, the chickens are slaughtered following the birth of the baby so that chicken soup, believed to be essential to healthy and abundant breastmilk production, can be made for the new mother.* Pilipino-Americans, especially in metropolitan areas, no longer practice this custom. Nevertheless, the belief in chicken soup as an important breastmilk stimulator often remains. A typical comment from our data exemplifies this, "If you plan to breastfeed (and most women do), you are given lots of soup after delivery."

Clearly, the diet arena provides great potential for conflict between Pilipino-American maternity patients and prenatal health care providers. Recent prenatal nutrition research argues for a greater weight gain than previously encouraged. Many nurses, midwives, and obstetricians now recommend women gain upwards of 30 pounds during pregnancy. Prescribing prenatal vitamin and mineral supplements is standard practice.

Our research data revealed that pregnant Pilipino-American

---

*Based on information supplied by nurse immigrants from the Philippines.

women are confused and upset by dietary practices, vitamin supplements, or drugs that contradict their country of origin values. Often shy, passive, and deferent, especially if they are new arrivals, and accustomed to showing respect to authority figures, Pilipino women rarely attempt to explain their dietary beliefs to the obstetrician and maternity nurses caring for them, according to our data. Their usual course of action is to politely concur with the prenatal dietary or drug instructions and then return home to follow traditional tenets. A housewife explained it this way:

> Pilipina women will not take any medications, because they feel if you take any while you're pregnant it may harm the baby. This goes along with vitamins. They say they're going to take them, and take them home, but they won't take them. They believe that any medication will harm the baby, and they're very scared of having an abnormal baby. If nurses would explain that it won't hurt the mother or baby, and that it is important for the mom or the baby to be healthy, they will take it. They need to understand this. Americans automatically understand that vitamins will make the health of the mother and baby better, but Pilipinas don't understand this or believe this.

Mother-Daughter Conflict: East versus West

An underlying dynamic should be clarified here. As suggested earlier, all pregnant women are highly influenced by their mothers or mother surrogate regarding beliefs and behaviors associated with childbearing. In cultures in which emancipation of the young adult occurs, such as in England, Canada, and the United States, mother's influence is considerably diluted. In Asian cultures, on the other hand, respect for ancestry takes precedence over emancipation. Women, particularly, may never sever childhood ties with their family of origin. Our data show that it is not unusual for several generations of Pilipino families to live either together or in surrounding homes, even after having immigrated to the United States. Adherence to mother's dictates is especially important regarding childbearing issues, as the previous mention of *vahina-hai* suggests. Therefore mother's doctrines regarding childbearing behavior, which have been internalized by the daughter since childhood and are constantly reinforced by mother's continued presence, take precedence over health providers' prenatal instructions. As we mentioned earlier, to most immigrants, all medications are strictly prohibited during pregnancy, including prenatal vitamins, as Pilipina women believe all foreign substances are potentially dangerous. Even professional Pilipino women cling tenaciously to native beliefs.

Although one Philippines-educated nurse with diabetes knew that the condition places a pregnant woman in a high-risk maternity category, when pregnant herself she refused to take insulin. In her words, "I'm going to control by diet . . . I don't want to take the insulin. My mother said, 'Don't take medicine, it's bad for the baby.'"

Our data revealed, however, that a toll is extracted by this conflict between traditional and modern doctrines. Some Pilipina women express a need to compromise the opposing camps, adhering to mother's doctrine (the safest route) while including portions of the Western doctrine in benign and nonessential matters. As one woman described it:

> It's hard, you know, I'm an American, and I want to do it the American way because it's better. But I get home and my mom says, "Oh no, you must do this and this!" So I do this at home but when the nurse asks me I say yes, I do what you say. I try to do both.

Many women express difficulty maintaining the facade for prenatal providers, since, from her point of view, to alienate the doctors and nurses would be an unthinkable embarrassment for themselves and the professionals as well. Somehow the doctrines must be mediated in an effort to accomplish safe passage for self and infant. Anxieties regarding safe passage germinate in these conflicting doctrines, since both doctrines command respect. Conflict of doctrines provides grist for the fear that the fetus may be damaged.

Family Support

Our data indicate that interaction between Pilipina women and Western health care providers often leads to support system conflict in the minds of the women. In the islands, childbearing is regarded as a family-centered event. Both nuclear and extended family cluster to provide protection, sanction, and support to the childbearing couple and neonate. Decisions about health care are never made by pregnant women alone. All health providers in the present study had observed family closeness among Pilipino-American families. Nurses of Pilipino extraction explain the depth of these ties. As one nurse put it:

> If patients think the family won't be able to visit, they worry about it all through the pregnancy. It's not just that they want the family there; the family *must* be there. Otherwise, it's not right. If the family is not there, you know, if they're back home, the friends must be allowed to come. We are very close.

Western prenatal care is geared to serve emancipated adult females. Women are expected to make decisions and speak in their own behalf. An extended family is generally not included in the process of prenatal care or labor and delivery. Clearly, such factors contribute to a sense of conflict for these women, and to an anxious feeling that the support system is not what it should be for her welfare and that of her child.

Another aspect of the custom of extended family presence is that, once pregnant, a Pilipina woman is given a great deal of extra consideration. In rural enclaves in the Philippines where the custom exists in its purest form, pregnant women are expected to do very little work inside the family and none outside the family throughout the childbearing year. Family members assume her chores, freeing her to attend fully to the important process of producing the succeeding generation. Such honor does not, however, extend to unmarried women. Such pregnancies are considered a severe stigma for the woman and her entire family, and an unmarried pregnant woman may be completely ostracised from family support.

Activity

Western health care professionals take a dim view of inactivity during pregnancy and postpartum. Unaware that the Pilipina sedentary style results from a cultural belief that inactivity constitutes a protection for the mother and child, Westerners label these women "lazy." Nurses of Pilipino ancestry, however, explain "We spoil them; it's good." When these women are forced to activity following delivery, they are unaware of the Western view that such activity is beneficial. The transplanted Pilipina interprets the professional's action as evidence of shaming:

> They think when the nurse does that, it's because they don't like them, and they feel ashamed. The nurse should explain that it's for their own good, and why.

In the United States, all adult family members must often serve as wage earners in order to support the large Pilipino family. the customarily low-paying jobs Pilipinos fill makes this necessary. The Asian maternity patients in the present study usually contributed to the family income. (We found a notable exception in armed service families, where the relatively high pay scale and benefits allowed the family to exist on the service-husband's salary.) Therefore, Pilipino-American women are frequently forced to forego the pampering and consideration custom dictates as their due, and this further adds to their sense of a deficient support system. A nurse from the Phillipines said:

Back home we all have maids. Only the very poorest don't have them. The family helps. Here, if a woman doesn't have a family, friends will help. But if everybody's working, you know, it's hard.

Conflicts regarding customs and expectations create a perplexing atmosphere for Pilipino-American childbearing women. Numerous dichotomous prescriptions concerning behavior and expectations emerged from interviews with the diverse respondents of the study. However, anxieties over welfare of the woman and her fetus in relation to diet and prenatal medications, and a prevailing sense of an insufficient support system, clearly comprised the primary sources of stress.

Interpersonal Style and Social Approach:
Unintentional Shaming

Acceptable styles of interpersonal behavior, including social approach, vary according to cultural prescription. No universal agreement regarding courteous behavior exists. Alienation results when styles differ widely, as subtle initial social amenities, essential for facilitating deeper communication, may be violated. The Pilipino interpersonal style, in many ways, diametrically opposes the American style. Pilipino-American maternity patients report feeling confused, alienated, and embarrassed by the conflict.

As Asians, people of the Philippines follow the Asian style of indirect communication. This style is rooted in an Asian respect for authority and for elders, and in passive-voiced deference to others (Orque, 1979). Many Pilipinos think that it is socially inappropriate to speak in a style that is confrontive, too direct or immodest, or that suggests intimacy prematurely. In general Pilipino politeness calls for an initial social approach that should not be businesslike in order to show evidence of interest and concern, as manifested in "small-talk." A major variable of the communication style is the cultural need to avoid shaming and embarrassment. An American-born student nurse whose parents came from the Philippines, said, "You never tell someone you don't like what they're doing. You tell someone else, and hope it will get back to them, because you don't want to shame the person."

In contrast, Western health care providers more often communicate in a direct, aggressive, and confrontive style. The prevailing approach of obstetrical nurses and physicians is relatively impersonal, efficient, and rapid. Small-talk may or may not be initiated by the health care professional, but it usually *follows* rather than precedes "business." Regardless, small-talk is rarely seen to be of much importance. An American-born Pilipina told us, "Americans are very business-like—they get down to business right away. Pilipinos like to exchange pleasantries first."

Perplexity on both sides results from this incongruence in interpersonal styles. Pilipina women interpret the direct, business-like approach of their American health providers as shaming. Direct questions about intimate topics, and a lack of superficial personal chit-chat, embarrasses them. The resulting anxiety they experience further erodes their sense of a caring support system, which is so essential to successful mastery of the psychological developmental tasks of pregnancy.

On the other side, Western health providers are frustrated by the passive Pilipina patient whom they interpret as polite, evasive, and difficult to teach or treat. One obstetrical nurse summed up her frustration in the phrase ". . . like talking to a smiling wall." Our data reveal that health providers, frustrated by a lack of communication and compliance, often resort to withdrawal tactics or to coercion that further escalates the spiral of shaming avoidance and shared avoidance. In subtle ways, such factors constitute disruptive stress.

Language Barriers

Although English speaking, Pilipino-Americans have difficulty with the language because of the great variety of American idioms and accents. A Pilipino-American physician said, "To us, a turkey is a big bird Americans eat at Thanksgiving, not a disagreeable person."

We found that prenatal Pilipina women frequently became so anxious by the confrontive communication style of the doctors and nurses that anxiety further impaired their language mastery. Cadence and voice tones make matters worse. An unfamiliar language sounds rapid to the listener. Harried health professionals often shout directions in passing, using a machine-gun-like delivery. In an effort to avoid shaming themselves, Pilipina women rarely ask for clarification or reveal their lack of understanding. Asked directly if they understand, their response is almost always, "yes." Since they learn English in the Philippines, a lack of understanding means to them that they didn't learn English well enough.

Language barriers, therefore, clearly add to a prevailing sense of anxiety and of disturbing stress that befalls Pilipino-American childbearing women in the U.S. Less a function of the actual language itself, the source of difficulty lies more with the variety of idioms, slang, euphemisms, and acronyms used by American nurses and physicians. Rapid speech further compounds the difficulty. The resulting stress is often experience as a further deficiency in the support system as already suggested. However, the stress of not understanding and not being understood can seriously diminish self-esteem and a sense of competency. In this way, conflicts with social approach and language can result in category-three stressors, that is, a woman's nagging perception that she is inadequate to the task of childbearing and mothering before her. A graduate student from the Philippines said:

> Pilipinos have this colonial mentality—everything American must be better. When we fail to live up to the ideal, we feel the fault is in ourselves. And shame, you know, is always reflected on the whole family. You're wrong, the whole family's disgraced. That's real failure!

To have failed both self and family lays the ground work for inadequacy in the vital role of mother and preserver of the family.

RECOMMENDATIONS

Difficulties of custom, approach, and language can be addressed in several ways. We suggest the following:

Custom

When two cultures are unaware of the other's belief system, communication is interpreted. According to our data, westerners were unaware of the cultural beliefs of Pilipino-Americans, while Pilipino-Americans were unaware of Western health beliefs. These Asians are willing to learn new customs, but they must understand the meaning the custom has for the health care provider.

At one San Francisco hospital, almost half the nursing staff is of Pilipino ancestry. Although quite willing to talk with the investigators, these nurses did not help to make nurses from other cultural groups aware of their own people's beliefs. We suggest that cultural information be passed along in the form of workshops, printed material, or informal conversations. Additionally, several San Francisco hospitals have instituted liberal visiting policies that allow for the extended family to follow their customary involvement in childbearing.

Approach

The desire of Pilipino-Americans for "more personal" health care may be addressed by using patients' names, noting individual differences, and engaging in "small-talk." These procedures require little time and effort but can serve as productive solutions to problems involving approach.

Language

Health professionals can solve the problem of language barriers quite effectively by avoiding slang, speaking slowly, and supplying pictures and printed material. Pilipino-Americans' command of the written word often exceeds their understanding of spoken English.

Approaching the whole family when seeking information or giving instruction can also be effective. Since compliance to health prescriptions involves a family decision, addressing the decision-making body has applicability.

In diverse ways, major points of cultural conflict regarding customs approach and language become subtle sources of the kinds of prenatal stress found to be most disruptive to the normal psychological developmental progression through childbearing. This research has documented the contributing antecedent and consequent variables for one cultural group. While variations could be anticipated in other cultures, we hypothesize that a similar picture would emerge.

In light of the vast number of culturally disparate childbearing women who receive prenatal care in the US, and with the emerging awareness of the critical nature of psychological factors to healthy birth and parenting, further attention to cultural conflict in prenatal health care seems warranted. Significant further study might specifically collect respondent data that documents when women of disparate cultures experience enough cultural conflict and resulting stress to hamper their achievement of psychological developmental tasks of childbearing.

In a broader sense, the Pilipino-American's desire for "more personal" health care may well be echoed by a majority of recipients of health care of all cultural varieties. Health care that protects the ego system and cultural heritage of the recipient seems desirable for patients of all ethnic backgrounds.

REFERENCES

Affonso, D. (1975). Response to pain in experience of labor in a specific culture in Hawaii. In A. L. Clark (Ed.), *Impact on culture and child-bearing and child-rearing.* Honolulu: University of Hawaii Press.

Affonso, D. (1978). The Filipino American. In A. L. Clark (Ed.), *Culture child-bearing health professionals,* Philadelphia: Davis.

Ballou, J. (1978). The significance of reconciliative themes in the psychology of pregnancy. *Bulletin of the Menninger Clinic, 42,* 383–413.

Benedek, T. (1956). Psychobiological aspects of mothering. *American Journal of Orthopsychiatry, 26,* 272–278.

Bibring, G. L. (1959). Some considerations of the psychological processes in pregnancy. *The Psychoanalytic Study of the Child, 16,* 113–121.

Bibring, G. L., Dwyer, T., Huntington, D., & Valenstein, A. (1961). A study of psychological processes in pregnancy and of the earliest mother-child relationship. *The Psychoanalytic Study of the Child, 14,* 9–71.

Caplan, G. (1961). *An approach to community mental health.* New York: Grune & Stratton.

Cohen, R. (1979). Maladaptation to pregnancy. *Seminars in Perinatology, 3,* 15–24.

Cohen, R. (1966). Pregnancy stress and maternal perceptions of infant endowment. *Journal of Mental Subnormality, 12,* 18–23.

Cranley, M. S. (1981). Development of a task for the measurement of maternal attachment during pregnancy. *Nursing Research, 30*(5), 281–284.

Crawford, M. (1968). Physiological and behavioral cues to disturbance in childbirth. *Bulletin of the Sloan Hospital for Women, 14,* 132–142.

Deutsch, H. (1945). *The psychology of women Volume 2.* New York: Grune & Stratton.

Duff, D. F., & Arthur, R. J. (1973). Between two worlds: Filipinos in the U.S. Navy. In S. Sue & N. N. Wagner (Eds.), *Asian-Americans: Psychological Perspectives.* Palo Alto, CA: Science & Behavior Books.

Glaser, B. G., & A. L. Strauss (1967). *The discovery of grounded theory.* Chicago: Aldine.

Gorsuch, R., & M. Key (1974). Abnormalities of pregnancy as a function of anxiety and life stress. *Psychosomatic Medicine, 36,* 352–362.

Helper, M. M., Cohen, R. L., Beiteman, E. T., & Eaton, L. (1968). Life-events and acceptance of pregnancy. *Journal of Psychosomatic Research, 12,* 183–188.

Hunt, C. L. (1954). Relationship of ethnic groups: Filipinos in the U.S. In C. L. Hunt, et al. (Eds.), *Sociology in the Philippine setting.* Manila: Alemars.

Jacono, F. L. (1969). *Growing up in Philippine barrio,* New York: Holt & Rinehart.

Kalish, R. A., & Yuen, S. Y. (1973). Americans of East Asian ancestry: Aging and the aged. In N. N. Wagner & S. Sue (Eds.), *Asian Americans: Psychological perspectives,* Palo Alto, CA: Science & Behavior Books.

Lederman, R., Lederman, E., Work, B., & McCann, D. (1978). Relationship of psychological factors in pregnancy to progress in labor. *Nursing Research, 28,* 94–97.

Lott, J. L. (1976). Migration of a mentality: The Filipino Community. *Social Casework, 57,* 165–172.

Maxwell, E. K. (1979). Modeling life: The dynamic relationship between elder modelers and their proteges. (Doctoral dissertation, University of California, San Francisco, 1979), *Dissertation Abstracts International, 39,* 7531A.

McDonald, R. (1968). The role of emotional factors in obstetrical complications: A review, *Psychosomatic Medicine, 30,* 222–243.

Norbeck, J. S. (1981). Social support: A model for clinical research and application. *Advances in Nursing Science, 3,* 43–59.

Norbeck, J. S., & Tilden, V. P. (1983). Psychological and social factors in complications of pregnancy: A prospective, multivariate approach. *Journal of Health and Social Behavior, 24,* 30–46.

Nuckolls, K., Cassell, J., & Kaplan, B. (1972). Psychosocial assets, life crisis and the prognosis of pregnancy. *American Journal of Epidemiology, 95,* 431–441.

Nydegger, W. F., & Nydegger, C. (1966). *Tarong: A Illocos barrio in the Philippines.* New York: Wiley.

Orque, M. (1979). An evaluation of a caucasian nursing student's home visiting program for culturally relevant care of Filipino families (Doctoral dissertation, University of San Francisco, 1979). *Dissertation Abstracts International, 40,* 677B.

Rubin, R. (1967). Attainment of the maternal role, Part 1 and Part 2. *Nursing Research, 16*(3–4), 237–245/342–346.

Rubin, R. (1976). Maternal tasks in pregnancy. *Journal of Advanced Nursing, 1,* 367–376.

Shereshefsky, P., & Yarrow, L. (1973). *Psychological aspects of a first pregnancy and early postnatal adaptation.* New York: Raven.

Shon, S. P. (1972). The Filipino community and mental health: A study of Filipino-Americans in Mental Health District V of San Francisco. *Program Information Series,* Community Mental Health Training Program, Langley Porter Neuropsychiatric Institute, University of California, San Francisco, 3 (5).

Stern, P. N. (1980). Grounded theory methodology: Its uses and processes. *Image, 12,* 20–23.

Stern, P. N., Allen, L. M., & Moxley, P. A. (1982). The nurse as grounded theorist: History process and uses. *Review of Journal of Philosophy and Social Science, 7,* 200–215.

Udderberg, N., & Fagerstrom, C. (1976). The deliveries of daughters of reproductively maladjusted mothers. *Journal of Psychosomatic Research, 20,* 223–229.

U.S. Bureau of the Census (1978). *Statistical abstract of the United States: 1978,* (99th edition), Washington, D.C.

A COMPARISON OF CULTURALLY APPROVED BEHAVIORS AND BELIEFS BETWEEN PILIPINA IMMIGRANT WOMEN, U.S.-BORN DOMINANT CULTURE WOMEN, AND WESTERN FEMALE NURSES OF THE SAN FRANCISCO BAY AREA: RELIGIOSITY OF HEALTH CARE

Phyllis Noerager Stern, DNS, RN, FAAN
Dalhousie University School of Nursing, Halifax, Nova Scotia

Data from 201 interviews and 400 hours of observation with a population consisting of Pilipino childbearing women, dominant culture women, and western nurses, all residing in the San Francisco Bay Area, indicate that all three groups base their health care on acquired beliefs. This supernatural approach to health care suggests a religiosity context that applies to all three groups studied.

The findings from the present study indicate that health care is influenced by the beliefs of providers as well as consumers. A religiosity context helps us understand the zeal with which health providers attempt to convert their clients.

The present study addresses the following research questions: In a comparison of selected, culturally approved behaviors and beliefs of Philippines-born American women, US-born women of the dominant culture, and western female nurses, which behaviors and beliefs interfere with the delivery of health care to Pilipina-American childbearing women; and which belief systems are compatible between dominant-culture women and nurses. This study also aims to determine which shared beliefs and behaviors serve to transcend cultural affiliation.

Tagalog, the national language of the Philippines, has no "F" sound; therefore, the spelling Pilipina or Pilipino used in this paper represents a more culturally sensitive representation than the more familiar Western version of Filipino or Filipina.

This paper appears in quite different form in the published Proceedings of the Sixth National Transcultural Nursing Conference, Salt Lake City: University of Utah Press, 1981. This study was supported in part by Faculty Development Grant #2-405231-09501, University of California, and by the Biomedical Research Support Branch, Division of Research Facilities and Resources, National Institutes of Health.

HEALTH CARE AND BELIEF SYSTEMS

Health care beliefs, like religious beliefs, tend to take on value-laden perspectives: there is a "right" and "wrong" of care. Like religion, health beliefs are held with tenacity. The current controversy over abortion makes this point quite clear: Opponents state their position in terms of right versus wrong, or good versus evil. Supporting arguments call upon supernatural powers for proof: God's will versus women's God-given right.

HISTORICAL PERSPECTIVES

Time influences culturally learned behaviors and beliefs for both westerners and Pilipinos. In a dynamic society such as the United States, and in an emerging nation like the Philippines, time factors influence health beliefs. For example, in the United States 10 or 20 years ago, paranoia resulting from belief in the germ as an evil force causing disease, resulted in the separation of families at the time of childbirth. This same belief even separated the skin of mother and babe through swaddling. Mothers were instructed to keep their babies securely wrapped in blankets during feeding so that germs would not be carried back to the nursery.

In the Philippines, health practices are undergoing radical revision. The recent immigrant may hold to a different set of beliefs than the immigrant of 5–10 years past. A young childbearing Pilipina immigrant eager to learn western ways may be coerced by elders in her community to adhere to old practices.

GEOGRAPHIC PERSPECTIVES

Like the United States, the Philippines occupy a considerable geographic area, and like the U.S., the country enjoys marked cultural diversity. To speak of a typical Pilipina gives an impression as erroneous as naming a typical American. However, some commonalities exist that provide clues for the outsider.

LITERATURE REVIEW, SAMPLE AND METHOD

Background

The Philippines consist of 7,100 islands. Ethnically and culturally, the people of the Philippines developed diversely under foreign domination. Mainly Malayan, the Pilipino racial mixture reflects the

Negreto Pygmies, and invasions of Indonesians, Chinese, Spanish, Americans, and more recently, Japanese. The Spanish, who dominated the Philippines from 1521 until 1898 unified the islands to Catholicism. The main contribution of 50 years of American domination was universal education. The Philippines gained independence in 1947.

Pilipino immigration to the U.S. now takes on the proportions of a major movement as Pilipinos immigrate to the U.S. at the rate of 38,000 a year (U.S. Bureau of the Census, 1978). Some 60,000 reside in the San Francisco Bay Area alone. The scope of this paper precludes a complete history of Pilipino immigration to the United States. We refer the reader to DeGarcia (1979), Orque (1979), and Parreno (1977).

Studies in Health Care

Despite the size of this ethnic minority, studies dealing with health care of transplanted Pilipinos are markedly lacking. Nursing studies that pertain to Pilipino childbearing in the United States include McKensie and Chrisman (1977), who discovered folk beliefs through a small interview sample, and Affonso's (1975), work on childbirth perceptions of 65 Pilipina women living in Hawaii. Norton (1980), working with pregnant Pilipinas in Seattle, found that these women consider customs of the Philippines to be "normal," and U.S. customs, "not normal." The present study is unique in its focus on the interaction between western health care professionals and Pilipina childbearing women in the United States. In a previous paper (1980), my co-investigators and I considered the difficulties for the transplanted Pilipina in accomplishing the psychological maturational process of pregnancy in a foreign culture. Another aspect of this study (1981), looks at problems of health teaching between Pilipina immigrants and western nurses. It was found in that part of the study that differences in beliefs concerning *approach, custom,* and *language* lead to a communication breakdown between the two groups.

METHOD AND SAMPLE

During 1978–1980 data were collected from seven San Francisco Bay Area health care facilities. Data consisted of 201 interviews and over 400 hours of observation. The original sample of 91 persons included 40 Pilipina-American, pregnant or postpartal women, 10 husbands, and 10 mothers of the women, and a racially-mixed sample of registered, vocational, and student nurses, aides, and

physicians. The professional group represented a wide age range.
Later interviews were conducted with 40 dominant-culture women
of childbearing age living in the Bay Area. It should be noted that
the Bay Area is somewhat unique in its cultural, ethnic, and sociological diversity, and that the opinions of these women, therefore,
may not be, and probably are not, nationally typical. The women
were caucasians, and religions origins fell into the groups of 40%
Catholic, 40% Protestant, 10% Jewish, and 10% "other." Western
nurses were observed in their natural work habitat, and some feedback from workshops based on earlier findings made up the balance of the data. Also, I asked Phillipines-born nurses about beliefs and behaviors of their home country. They acted as chief
informants.

Data were analyzed using grounded theory, a modified form of
field method developed by Glaser and Strauss (1967). This method
aims to discover salient variables in a social scene rather than testing
hypotheses gleaned from other theories. In overlapping processes of
data collection, coding, categorizing, conceptualizing, reducing, re-
sampling, and theoretical coding, constructs emerge that identify the
main problems from the actors' viewpoint, and what the actors
do to solve those problems (Glaser, 1978; Maxwell & Maxwell, 1980;
Stern, 1980; Stern, Allen, & Moxley, 1982; Schatzman & Strauss,
1973; and Wilson, 1977).

Developing a Theoretical Construct: Religiosity
of Health Care

During presentations of earlier portions of this work, I emphasized
the difference between belief and ideation: one can challenge ideas,
but rational arguments have little effect of belief systems. I reflected
on the change in health care beliefs (claimed to be based on
"science") in my own professional lifetime. However, it was after
hearing two nurses, both possessing advanced academic degrees, argu-
ing over the abortion issue using passion for support rather than
logic, that the theoretical notion of health care as a religious endeavor struck me. Using the data and findings from the earlier parts
of the study, I hypothesized that health care beliefs take on a
religious quality. When beliefs originate from our own health culture,
we call them science, and they become *truths.* Foreign beliefs we call
superstition, and we label them *false beliefs.*

Having formed this hypothesis of religiosity in health care, I followed the ground rules of grounded theory and collected more data
to support or refute this construct, and to define the limits of the

variable, the conditions under which it occurs, and the outcomes of its existence or absence.

FINDINGS

Part 1 of the findings includes comparisons between the three groups that center around the variables of social interaction, family closeness displays, community concern displays, sexual displays, and pregnancy reaction: health versus illness. Part 2 discusses converging variables that transcend the three groups.

PART 1: DIVERGING BELIEFS

Social Interaction

Variation occurred between the three groups in beliefs involving communication, courtesy, and autonomy. Interactionally, the Pilipinas we observed practiced the Asian style of indirect communication and nonconfrontation. As an example, if "A" has a problem with "B," she tells "C" about it and hopes it will get back. In our study group, confrontation was considered the height of rudeness reflecting shame on the confrontor, the confrontee, and the families of both. Pilipinos in our study considered it polite to engage in "small-talk" before business. Newly arrived immigrants complain that Americans are "all business." The literature describes Pilipinas as deferring and dependent. It was found that length of residence in the United States, and district of origin limits this variable. Ilicionos from from the northern Philippines pride themselves on their business-like personalities, and other immigrants become more assertive, "as soon as we learn your ways."

Western dominant culture women were found to be moderately direct. In business matters they reported that they were "learning to speak up." The conditions that limited this variable were a "touchy subject" that led to less directness, and in the other extreme, feelings of anger and injustice that allowed them to be more confronting. They rarely engaged in "small talk" while doing business. Dominant-culture women like making their own decision, but generally consulted family and friends on important issues.

Western nurses in our data were taught to communicate directly, and to face an issue "straight on." They stated a belief in confrontation. However, we did observe nurses discussing *other* nurses with whom they were having problems behind their backs.

In interacting with patients, nurses were called "impersonal" by the other two groups. Patients in both groups could recall individual nurses who had taken the time to treat them as "persons," but said that, in general, hospital workers presented a "business-like" persona. Nurses were seen as being "too busy" to engage in "small talk," and nurses themselves said they would "chat" with a patient only rarely. Nurses expected their women patients to make independent decisions.

Pilipinas object to vulgar language. Several Pilipina women in this study complained about nurses who used swear words and obscenities in their presence.

Family Closeness Displays

Behaviors investigated in this category included respect for elders, respect for parents, deference to husband, and assistance to the child-rearing family. As befitting beliefs in ancestor worship, Pilipinos we talked with were taught to treat their parents with respect. Respect for elders, in general, and for authority figures was encouraged as well. Given this training, Pilipinas find it extremely difficult to complain about hospital care.

Nuclear and extended Pilipino families in this study maintained close ties, and often lived in the same house together. The birth of a baby became sanctified only after friends and family viewed the new arrival. Following birth, new parents spent months with relatives or friends who shared in the work of childrearing to "give them a good start." Deference to one's husband was the culturally-approved norm, but as a group of Pilipinas told me, "That's the way the men think it is, but that's not the way it really is."

Dominant culture women expressed a philosophical concern for the plight of old people, but few spent actual time helping this age group. They all expressed a belief in being independent and living apart from parents and in-laws. Many spoke of adolescent rebellion as appropriate behavior.

The dominant culture group viewed themselves as sharing decision-making with their spouse or lover, a sort of "win-a-few-lose-a-few" proposition. Family help following childbirth generally consisted of a week-long visit by the woman's mother.

Nurses displayed a respect for youth, giving more attention to young primiparas than older primiparas or multiparas. They displayed little concern for the importance of the patient's ties with older relatives, grandparents, aunts, older friends, or the concern these relatives might have for the patient.

Nurses in this study uniformly encouraged emancipation. There seemed to be no question about the "right way" of an adult woman living apart from parents. Philippines-born nurses did not share this view.

The nurses in this study expressed proliberation views. They spoke of the importance of the "couple bond," but, as above, they expected their patients to make independent decisions.

Following birth, the hospital nurses in this study felt released from responsibility for the patient's care, although in some cases a single home visit by the public health nurse was arranged.

We discovered an outstanding case of counter-conversion in the matter of family presence. In one San Francisco hospital, a western-born maternity supervisor, aware of the need for open visiting by family and extended family to the postpartal Pilipina, arranged for open ward visiting. Although the rules were changed to accommodate Pilipinos, dominant culture patients enjoyed this open visiting as well.

Concern for Community

Hospitality emerged as the variable indicative of community concern. We found a wide variation between the three groups.

Pilipinas in this study professed and displayed strong ties to, and influence by, their community. Their hospitality to one another, as described by one woman, "reaches ridiculous proportions." Commonly a Pilipino family opens its home to new immigrants who may be absolute strangers. The newcomers stay on for months or years until they can strike out for themselves.

In California, in general, and the Bay Area in particular, socially correct behavior takes on definite reserve in the matter of hospitality. One telephones before visiting, and permission to intrude upon another's privacy is either granted or refused according to the convenience of the host. This is known locally as "protecting your space." Data revealed that variations in the ritual phone call category occur when friends are close enough so that, "I can say it's not a good time to visit." The other condition that affects the category lies in length of residence in California. Newer arrivals were found to favor hospitable social interactions.

The word "hospitable" was absent from descriptions of nurses. Nurses, as in the interaction category above, were seen by the other two groups as business-like and impersonal.

Sexual Displays

Wide differences exist between Pilipinas and the other two groups in the categories of chastity, physical modesty, public displays of affections, and sex choice of physician. Information gathered on Pilipinas gives direction for student assignment and risk assessment.

Pilipinas are expected to retain their virginity until marriage. This strongly held belief leads to withdrawal of support by families and whole communities from an unmarried pregnant Pilipina, thus placing her in a high-risk category.

Pilipinas report extreme physical modesty. I was told that half the physicians in the Philippines are women, because no Pilipina would allow herself to be examined by a male doctor. This has implications for student assignment: I would now assign only female students to the physical care of Pilipinas.

In public, Pilipinos considered it appropriate for members of the same sex to display affections. Males may hold hands with males, females with females. Heterosexual sex displays, however, are tabu in public.

All but two of the dominant-culture women considered virginal marriage passé. The two exceptions cited religiosity as a basis for their opinion. All women questioned "minded" being examined by a male physician, but only 8 out of 40 women selected a woman gynecologist. The exception again were Pilipina nurses.

We observed western nurses engaging in flirtatious behavior with persons of the opposite sex—usually physicians. Sometimes the patients suffered neglect due to this dalliance. Conversation in the delivery room, for example, strayed away from patient's concerns to flirtatious exchanges.

Pregnancy Reaction: Health-Illness

We found a sharp dichotomy between Pilipinas and the other two groups in the point of view of the pregnant woman as a fragile being. Pilipinas see pregnancy as a time for inactivity, and a time to be cared for. The same belief holds true for the weeks following birth.

Both nurses and western women viewed pregnancy as a healthy normal time for women. Both groups believed in exercise as the pathway to greater well-being. The comparisons described in part one are represented in Figure 1.

PART 2: CONVERGING BELIEFS

Data indicate shared beliefs between the three groups that give clues for crossing cultural barriers. Converging beliefs involved science, education, humor, family influence, and avoiding shame.

All three groups (albeit with certain reservations) believed in the

Behaviour / Belief	Pilipinas	Western Women	Western Nurses
SOCIAL INTERACTION	**ASIAN**	**WESTERN**	**HEALTH CULTURE**
Communication	Indirect	Mod Direct	Overt Directness
	⌒--⌒	⌒∿⌒	⟩ Straight on ⟩ (Covertly indirect)
Confrontation	Non-confronting	Mod Confronting	Confronting
Personal/Impersonal	Personal (social) (Small talk)	Business-like (Some small talk)	Impersonal (No small talk)
Autonomy	Dependent/Independent	Mod Independent	Pro-independence
FAMILY CLOSENESS DISPLAYS	**OVERT**	**COVERT**	**LOW PRIORITY**
Respect - elders	Ancester worship	Weak	Respect youth
Parents	Respect	Rebellion	Pro Emancipation
Husband	Overt deference Covert decisions	Co-equal	Pro Liberation
Helping new parents	Live with elders	Grandmother 1 week	Dropped
CONCERN FOR COMMUNITY	**STRONG**	**WEAK**	**WEAK**
Hospitality	Strong	As convenient	Official Business
SEXUAL DISPLAYS	**MODEST**	**LAISSEZ-FAIRE**	**BOLD LANGUAGE**
Chastity: Sex and Language	Chaste in both	Experimental in both	Activity ?
Physical modesty	Overt	Covert	Covert
Public Affection	Same sex OK	Opposite sex OK	Flirtatious - opposite sex
Physician Sex choice	Female	Male	Male
PREGNANCY REACTION	**FRAGILITY**	**STRENGTH**	**STRENGTH**
Health / Illness	Illness	Health	Health
Activity / Inactivity	Inactivity	Activity	Activity

Figure 1. Comparison of culturally approved behaviors and beliefs between immigrant Pilipinas, western women, and western nurses.

miracle of science. Modern health care in the Philippines is based on the American model and the newest hospitals rival our own in technology.

All three groups valued education. Given the right approach, the nurse finds Pilipinas as well as western women eager to learn.

Transcultural humor was seen to exist. Joking and response occurred between the three groups.

All three groups admitted to the influence of family and social network on the individual. Nurses and dominant culture women often saw the influence as negative: "Father made me an over-achiever," or "She has this schizophrenogenic mother." Pilipinas only spoke of the positive influence of their family.

All women in this study felt a need to avoid shame in social interactions. Pilipinas avoided shame by pretending to understand when they did not. This was often true of western women too, " I didn't understand a word the doctor told me, but I didn't want him to think I was stupid." Nurses tended to avoid the shame of not getting through to Pilipinas. They would walk away from a problem rather than suffer the humiliation of being a poor teacher.

CONCLUSIONS

Health care based on beliefs, expressed here as religiosity, become clear in this study comparing nurses, western women, and Pilipina immigrants. We may simply have different dogma or "right way" that we worship. Other authors, most notably Mendelson (1980), have suggested that health care takes on the religious mantle of supernaturalness.

Religiosity extends to other fields of care. Belief-based treatment guides care of the cancer patient. The prevailing belief in mutilation surgery over quality of life now undergoes question.

One hesitates mentioning psychiatry, because some already regard that field as witchcraft. However, recent papers suggest that mental health care can legitimately take place within the framework of the culturally different patient's belief system (Walthers, 1977; Warner, 1977). These papers support the notion that it is what one believes that counts.

Viewing health care as a religious endeavor gives us a clearer understanding of the tenuousness of our beliefs of "right" and "wrong" treatment. Tomorrow we may convert to beliefs of health care that today seem nonscientific and heretical.

REFERENCES

Affonso, D. (1975). Response to pain in the experience of labor in a specific culture in Hawaii. In L. A. Clark (Ed.), *Impact of Culture and Childbearing and Childrearing,* Honolulu: University of Hawaii Press.

DeGarcia, R. T. (1979). Perspectives on the Asian American's implications for health care. *Washington State Journal of Nursing, special supplement,* 9–19.

Glaser, B. G. (1978). *Theoretical sensitivity.* Mill Valley, CA: Sociology Press.

Glaser, B., & Strauss, A. (1967). *The discovery of grounded theory.* Chicago: Aldine.

Maxwell, E. K., & Maxwell, R. J. (1980). Search and research in ethnology: Continuous comparative analysis. *Behavior Science Research, 15,* 219–243.

Mendelson, R. S. (1980). *Confessions of a medical heretic.* Chicago: Warner.

McKensie, J. L., & Chrisman, N. J. (1977). Healing herbs, gods, and magic: Folk health beliefs among Filipino-Americans. *Nursing Outlook, 25,* 326–329.

Norton, S. M. (1980). A descriptive study of the postpartum health beliefs and practices of selected pregnant Filipino women. Unpublished Masters thesis, University of Washington.

Orque, M. (1983). *Ethnic nursing care: A multicultural approach.* St. Louis: Mosby.

Orque, M. (1979). An evaluation of a Caucasian nursing student's home visiting program for culturally relevant care of Filipino families. (Doctoral dissertation, University of San Francisco, 1979). *Dissertation Abstracts International,* Order No. 7918665.

Parreno, H. (1977). How Pilipinos deal with stress. *Washington State Journal of Nursing, Winter,* 3–6.

Schatzman, L., & Strauss, A. L. (1973). *Field research.* Englewood Cliffs, NJ: Prentice-Hall.

Stern, P. N. (1981). Solving problems of cross-cultural health teaching: The Filipino childbearing family. *Image, 13,* 47–50.

Stern, P. N. (1980). Grounded theory methodology: Its uses and processes. *Image, 12,* 29–33.

Stern, P. N., Allen, L. M., & Moxley, P. A. (1982). The nurse as grounded theorist: History processes and uses. *The Review Journal of Philosophy and Social Science, 7,* 200–215.

Stern, P. N., Tilden, V. P., & Maxwell, E. (1980). Culturally induced stress during childbearing: The Pilipino-American experience. *Issues in the Health Care of Women, 2*(3–4), 67–81.

U.S. Bureau of the Census (1978). *Statistical abstract of the United States:* (99th edition). Washington, DC.

Walthers, W. E. (1977). Community psychiatry in Tutuila, American Samoa. *American Journal of Psychiatry, 134,* 917–919.

Warner, R. (1977). Witchcraft and soul loss: Implications for community psychiatry. *Hospital and Community Psychiatry, 28,* 686–690.

Wilson, H. S. (1977). Limiting intrusion—Social control of outsiders in a healing community. *Nursing Research, 26,* 103–110.

CULTURE SHOCK AND THE WORKING WOMAN: SURVIVING WEST COAST TO NORTHERN LOUISIANA RELOCATION

Phyllis Noerager Stern, DNS, RN, FAAN
Dalhousie University School of Nursing, Halifax, Nova Scotia

Mary Eve Baskerville Cousins, MSN, RN
Louisiana State University Medical School, Shreveport, Louisiana

Women in highly specialized professions often find relocation, with its concomitant culture shock, a necessity for maximum career advancement. An insider's view of culture shock derived from participant observation data suggests that sociocultural and mechanical differences may be overcome through personal qualities of egregiousness, a portable support system, and a penchant for self-actualization. Social interactional factors aiding the transition include neighborliness, having options, and showing respect. Unresolved culture shock may result in ghettoism or cultural identity crisis.

As more women mount career ladders, they come to realize that rapid assent often requires moving to another part of their country or another part of the world. To rise to the top of their profession, women as well as men, must go where the opportunities are. Women who once trailed willingly or unwillingly behind their men, moving for career reasons, have come to understand the other side of relocation, and its concomitant culture shock. That is, these women must learn to accommodate to the new culture of the workplace as well as the culture shock of new sights, new people, new accents, and new schools for the children.

This chapter was written when the senior author was Professor and Coordinator of Graduate Studies in Maternal-Child and Family Nursing at The College of Nursing, Northwestern State University, Shreveport, Louisiana. The concepts in this chapter were presented in a different form to the Seventh Annual Transcultural Nursing Conference, Seattle, Washington, September 1, 1981, and appears in their printed proceedings.

Grateful acknowledgement is extended to the Master of Science in Nursing and the Bachelor of Science in Nursing Students of Northwestern State University for their helpful suggestions in the preparation of the manuscript.

This chapter tells the story of one professional woman who successfully overcame the culture shock of relocation. The processes, stressors, phases, and characteristics of the actors are described in considerable detail. The reasons for this are twofold: to help the woman contemplating a move to experience anticipatory socialization, and to support the mental health of the women in culture shock by suggesting that she will survive.

Because the authors are nurses, it was natural for them to apply life experience to patient care. Therefore, the implications beyond the study have to do with the culture shock of patients entering the new environment of health care, where they find new sights, new people, new accents, and where they pretty much leave their families back in their other world.

Use of first person within this paper represents the voice of the senior author whose story it tells. The second author participated in the collection and analysis of data and in the preparation of the final manuscript.

This study addresses the research question: What variables are pivotal to surviving and resolving the culture shock of relocation. My comparison of the subcultures of two United States provinces, the San Francisco Bay Area and northern Louisiana, points to the contrast between the two settings and provides the basis for the discovery of major cultural shockers. The process of overcoming cultural shock is presented within a trajectory of four phases. Social and personal factors that contribute to a positive outcome are described, alternate outcomes are discussed, and transcultural health care implications are addressed.

PURPOSE OF THE STUDY

The importance of this study lies within the following reasons: (a) the descriptive, subjective experiences and feelings of the investigator may bring alive for the listener the intensity of the upheaval and trauma lived through by the person in culture shock; (b) as Stouffer (1955/1966) points out, culture shock can have an educational and broadening impact; (c) the factors that aided in a positive resolution of culture shock may be applied as well to other situations where culture shock is a problem, as in the case of nurses moving from one institution to another; and (d) these same factors may support patients entering the shockingly different culture of the health-care system.

BACKGROUND

Culture has been described by Olien (1978) as a system, and by Tylor (1871/1958) as a complex whole encompassing knowledge, beliefs, art, morals, law, and custom. A number of authors, generally anthropologists visiting foreign countries, have described culture shock. Oberg (1954), for example, describes culture shock as a condition that occurs when all the patterns and rules governing social behavior are replaced. Brein and David (1971) attribute culture shock to the breakdown of interpersonal communication between interactions from different cultures. Culture shock is characterized by such feelings as confusion, alienation, hostility, and anxiety (Taft, 1976). It has been described by Lundstedt (1963) as "a form of personality maladjustment . . . with subjective feelings of loss, and a sense of isolation and loneliness" (p. 3). Alvin Toffler (1970) compares the condition to that of a soldier in combat or the person who has experienced disaster. According to Toffler, "first we find the same evidences of confusion, disorientation, or distortion of reality. Second, there are the same signs of fatigue, anxiety, tenseness, or extreme irritability. Third, in all cases, there appears to be a point of no return—a point at which apathy and withdrawal set in . . . in short, the available evidence strongly suggests that over stimulation" (that is, sensory overload) "may lead to bizarre and anti-adaptive behavior" (p. 309).

Toffler's description made me feel somewhat relieved that my own shocky reaction fell within a paradigm of normalcy. My own description of culture shock relates to the senses. The geography, typology, and demography of northern Louisiana seemed the real-life version of Burt Reynolds' movie "Smokey and the Bandit." Here in Louisiana were the country roads, the bald cypress standing knee-deep in bayou water, the pickup trucks, and here and there, the "good ole' boys" wearing plastic mesh baseball caps. For a stranger to take up residence in a place seen before only in films, brought forth hair-tingling feelings of unreality. "Good lord," I thought, "I'm living in a movie." This was clearly a distortion of reality of the kind Toffler described. Although I subscribed to the local newspaper 3 months prior to moving, and did a fair amount of reading about the area, no amount of preparation softens the blow of culture shock. No matter what you do, it happens. I would like to add here that my work place in California was located in San Francisco, however, I made my home in a suburban area 30 miles south of the city. In Louisiana, I worked in the city, but lived in a semirural area 10 miles from the downtown area of Shreveport.

The culture shock patients experience is similar. Ramsden (1980), writing in *Physical Therapy,* describes the situation. A serious problem, according to Ramsden, is the unstated "rules" that one learns only by breaking them. "The 'rules' governing professional behavior, known and adhered to by the care-givers, are rarely made explicit to the patients" (p. 290). The same may be said of the rules of an alien culture. For some time, rules remain hidden and amorphous.

However, as Stouffer (1955/1966) points out, from culture shock comes an opportunity for learning, for broadening one's horizons, and, I might add, for achieving a sense of mastery. The main thrust of this paper then, is the positive resolution of culture shock.

METHOD

Sample

Field notes contain data from a 12-month period of participant observation from August, 1980 through August, 1981. Collection sights in Louisiana include the cities of Shreveport, Bossier, Minden, Natchitoches, and Alexandria. Institutions include a college of nursing, a rural university campus, a large medical school, and six community hospitals. Subjects include nursing and medical educators, practitioners and students, clients and lay persons. Documents such as handbooks, newspapers, and other printed material make up the remainder of the data.

Analysis

Data were analyzed using the constant comparison method of grounded theory (Glaser & Strauss, 1967). In this way, the conceptual framework was derived from the data (Stern, 1980). Coded data were clustered into naturally related categories, and compared categories were then linked and reduced until variables that explained important processes in the setting emerged. Major variables were then compared with those of other theorists in the field. During the last 2 months of the study, a number of additional interviews were conducted to determine the validity of the findings, for ". . . as Goodenough suggests, an analysis which does not ring true to the natives is immediately suspect . . ." (Feinburg, 1979, p. 546). Similarly, findings from this study presented to southern audiences underwent further analysis on this account.

FINDINGS

Comparison of Settings

In this report, I compare San Francisco and the Bay Area with Shreveport and the north Louisiana countryside that surrounds it. I suggest that no two cities in North America are so different as these, although like comparisons might be drawn between Anchorage and New Orleans, or Halifax and Calgary. San Francisco, where my family had lived for three generations, is semidesert because of its short yearly rainfall. It is cooled by ocean and bay fogs, making fall clothing year-round attire. Steep dry hills afford vistas of great distance, and native trees and shrubs grow dark leaves, a protection against arid conditions. Although we may say that no archetypical citizen of a city exists, San Franciscans and Bay Area dwellers in general pride themselves on the permissiveness of their culture. Even though it is a business center, offering services as the chief commodity, the natives place great emphasis on self-actualization. An opening conversational gambit might be, "What are you into?" Meaning yoga, meditation, jogging, or the like. As a major coastal city with a population of 680,700 (San Francisco, California Chamber of Commerce, personal communication, August 21, 1981), San Francisco is cosmopolitan in nature, and the citizens are generally tolerant of what would seem to north Louisianians unusual and strange.

Shreveport by contrast can be considered semitropical. Ample rains and warm summer temperatures make air conditioning necessary about 6 months of the year. Situated in the northwest corner of Louisiana, Shreveport spreads westward from the banks of the Red River. The relatively flat terrain boasts lush vegetation, and almost year-round blooms. Colorful birds brighten barren winter months. Although, again, no typical citizen exists, Shreveporters and north Louisianians in general pride themselves on their conservatism. Families stay on there for generations, and have a sense of history about the place. Married women are often asked, "Who *were* you?" Shreveport, with a population of 205,342 (Shreveport, Louisiana Chamber of Commerce, personal communication, August 21, 1981) is a trade center. The chief commodity is services. Natives place great emphasis on the importance of the total person, and a typical opening conversational gambit might be, "What church do ya'll belong to?" For all its stability, Shreveporters are remarkably tolerant of what would seem to San Franciscans unusual and strange.

Categories of Stressors

The following cursory description of stressors is designed to give the reader a sense of Shreveport and the north Louisiana region, and the things surprising to *me*. A more detailed description of the area may find its way into a future paper, perhaps patterned after Glittenberg's study of Brekenridge (1981).

The pattern for this analysis originated with Oberg (1954) and was later refined by Brink and Saunders (1976). Modifications have been made for a better fit with the present data.

Mechanical Differences

In the initial stages of shock, the mystery of which things are dangerous and which things are not dangerous is overwhelming. From the distance of a year, dangers seen in the Shreveport area retreated into mere differences from San Francisco. The main dissimilarities involve services, water supply, trash, and roads. To the Californian, certain services within the metropolitan area of Shreveport are remarkably inefficient; utilities, for instance, often fail. Some services, on the other hand, are available to all but poverty-level persons: maid service for example. Only upper-middle class persons in California have maids as a rule. Louisiana has been named—by Louisianians—"The trash capital of the world," and litter lines the roadways. Trash even contaminates the water supply in some areas; however, there are movements to amend these conditions. The water that serves San Francisco, piped in from the Sierra mountains, is stored in Crystal Springs Lake. The lake is fenced and fishing, boating, and swimming is prohibited. A major freeway was turned away from its shores by an angry clamor from the citizenry.

Runoff, and water from Black Bayou fills Cross Lake, Shreveport's reservoir. Cross Lake offers an ideal fishing site for bass, catfish, and bream. Fish bait, often live crickets, can be bought in styrofoam containers which are then often discarded along the shore and in the inlets. Although swimming is prohibited, the exhaust from water-skiing boats, and oil from cans tossed overboard cause the lake surface to be coated with an oily slick. The shores of Cross Lake are sprayed regularly with malathion in an effort to retard the growth of mosquitoes. A neighbor's septic tank drained into the lake, but this caused him little concern because, "mine isn't the only one and anyway they use so many chemicals, it could kill anything. Besides, we have a well." Mind you, the area does have its environmentalists. The construction of a freeway over the lake was delayed for several years because of their protests, but now, building proceeds. This, however, seems to be a nationwide trend.

California boasts an elaborate freeway system. Louisiana has few. Dead creatures on the roads of each state give another clue to the differences in animal inhabitants of the two environments. Jogging down California streets, one finds the odd dead cat, dog, bird, or squirrel. Running down a Louisiana road, one finds dead dogs, armadillos, turtles, toads, frogs, and snakes.

Customs

Disparity in food, clothing, and family closeness appeared most consistently in the data. Both settings pride themselves on the quality of local fish: multiple varieties in California; catfish is the speciality of north Louisiana. I have said, and have elicited a chuckle from the natives (so I guess it's okay to say), "in north Louisiana, folks will eat anything, as long as it's deep fried." This can be compared with a favorite Japanese dish found on the west coast, *tempura,* which consists of fried shrimp and vegetables. Although the stereotypical statement about fried foods ignores the nuances of the situation, locals (even some health professionals) confess to a fondness for what they call, "good greasy food." It is sort of a joke on themselves—they know better, but it tastes *so good.*

Middle class Shreveporters and north Louisianians embrace current American trends in dress. However, they insist that the garments be constructed of polyester. Reasons for choice of this fabric can be easily understood. As one citizen put it, "the greatest thing that ever happened to this country was the invention of the wash and wear suit—before that we used to look like we slept in our clothes." San Franciscans, on the other hand, favor natural fibers. As trendsetting San Francisco haberdasher Wilks Bashford says, "you have to learn to love the wrinkles."

Northern Louisianians maintain close family ties. Families commonly exchange meals several times a week. Children are valued. Bay Area dominant culture women on the other hand, express "a belief in being independent and living apart from parents and inlaws" (Stern, 1981, p. 90).

Communication

The classic line that sums up communication differences was directed to my husband and me by our local banker, "you have an accent, where ya'll from?" On the west coast, "ya'll" translates to "you guys," a unisex term. And I might add that I never spoke with an accent before; *other* people had accents. The suddenness with which I acquired one seemed like magic. Some communication difficulties did not surface until the period of shock was beginning to resolve. In culture shock, it is *what you don't know that you don't know* that causes the anguish.

Belief Systems

Natives of north Louisiana generally hold church, graciousness, and protection of property in high regard. Shreveport itself is a city of many churches, all of them well attended. Blue laws are observed, and although one can buy a pound of butter on Sunday, one may not buy a butter dish.

Natives prize courtesy and hospitality. They despair of someone who is "too busy to be polite." In contrast to their gentility, most households contain one or two guns in working order for the purpose of "protecting" their property. One of my neighbors owned five.

Most Bay Area residents attend church sporadically. Few own firearms except for hunting purposes and "protecting their space" is seen as more important than graciousness.

Social Order

To the observer, the social order of Northern Louisiana is marked by stability. The citizenry are reluctant to give up old standards. Examples of race differentiation and the position of women in the social scheme illustrate this point. Few natives confessed to a belief in the superiority of white persons over black. However, to the observer, the separation of the races seems quite exact, particularly in regard to housing and education. One rarely attends a social gathering of mixed racial guests. The sight of a mixed couple is extremely rare. When I jogged down the road, black people fishing by the lake never spoke unless addressed directly. This was strikingly different from California, where joggers are fair game for the side-of-the-road commentary that is considered part of the social norm.

Many nurses expressed concern over the social situation of race separation suggesting that this impeded the development of a trusting relationship between themselves and their black clients. However, as Durkheim (1915, 1930, 1947) points out, society structures the actions of the individual; therefore, these nurses felt powerless to effect change in the existing social system.

The majority of San Francisco women support feminist ideologies. By contrast, home and family are the stated priorities of northern Louisiana women. Forced heirship laws persist. In Louisiana, one's child inherits a percentage of a parent's property regardless of the financial need of surviving spouse or child. I learned about women's view of their station in the family when I began to ask about Yankees. "Yankee women are pushy," I was told, "and their husbands are henpecked." I am not considered a Yankee, incidentally; Californians are committed to some kind of separate category by north Louisianians.

PHASES OF SHOCK

The following description of the phases in my cultural shock may differ somewhat from those of other authors. For example, I experienced no honeymoon phase, but instead, plunged immediately into the stage of acute shock. The honeymoon phase along with the phase of enculturation or "going native" are described by Brink and Sanders (1976), but are not substantiated by my personal experience or by the data collected at the time of this writing.

Acute Shock

This phase, which lasts the usual crisis period of from 6–8 weeks, is marked by disorientation, anxiety, grief, and extreme paranoia. One simply does not know whom or what to trust. I had moved before, but I always had the old family home to which I knew I could return. Now my home was sold and slated for destruction. Toffler (1970) describes home as follows: "In a harsh, hungry and dangerous world, home, even when no more than a hovel, came to be regarded as the ultimate retreat, rooted in the earth, handed down from generation to generation, one's link with both nature and the past" (p. 83). My California home had been in the family for 55 years and many ghosts lived there.

My shock was made more profound by the philosophy of the work place. At the University of California, San Francisco, the stated philosophy is publish or perish. In this phase of extreme shock, it seemed to me that the unstated philosophy of my new setting was, a good teacher *teaches*. Even though this perception may have been colored somewhat by the distorted reality of acute shock, it seemed to me that my previously learned strategies for success became suddenly inappropriate.

Certain events fanned the flame of paranoia. My husband and I were burglarized, vandalized, cheated, and one of our windows was shot out. The initial phase began to resolve when I became sufficiently in touch with reality to understand that I had been in this area less than 2 months. My knowledge of crisis theory allowed me to begin to intellectualize—a useful coping strategy in some situations. (When all else fails, do a study of the problem.)

Making It Work

This phase, which Oberg (1954) calls beginning resolution, lasted over the next 4 months. For me, it was a time of trying out the new environment and looking for successes. In other words, seeing how much of Phyllis the natives could tolerate. Early in my residency, a clerk in my favorite bookstore told me, "if you're going to break the rules in this town, do it *real* big—then people will respect you." I followed her advice. As I mentioned earlier, north Louisianians are amazingly tolerant of the "strange and different." Students found the California extraterrestrial being entertaining. I began presenting papers around town, I made friends with the local science editor, and got a half page write-up and my picture in the paper.

During this time, prestigious friends from home visited, which added to the image I attempted to create—and then live up to. As I sped down the country roads in my nifty new sports car, I began to think, "hey, this ain't so bad."

Reappraisal

This phase is characterized by backlash. Suddenly, the glaring faults that *every* community has, became apparent. Although I had found a goodly number of the natives with whom I felt "in tune," and although my standard of living was infinitely better than it had been in my home state, the poverty, poor health, and obstacles to health care met by members of the lower classes distressed me endlessly. The movie I had been acting in became real life. This period occurred for me at 9 months postmove. I weighed successes with compromises. Is it possible, I wondered, to overlook ideological differences in favor of a richer life?

Resolving the Conflict

After approximately one year, I found myself getting on a plane for Shreveport after 4 days in San Francisco (my first trip back there since the move), and realizing with a start that I was glad to be going home—to *Shreveport!* Resolution of the shock of living in an alien culture takes a variety of forms that come under the category of *having options.* Beiser and Collomb (1981) point to ". . . the ability to creatively integrate elements of the old and new cultures" (p.

1352) as a factor that makes for a successful transition. Certainly southerners had much to teach me about graciousness and hospitality, and for my part, I realized that I need not give up trying for professional success. I had the option too of working to change the ideological differences I could not abide. This action, in truth, enhanced my professional success. Having a choice to opt out or relocate somehow facilitated resolution. Less favorable resolutions can result from being denied the option of leaving the scene: (a) ghettoism, that is, remaining aloof from the mainstream; and (b) prolonged cultural identity crisis, never belonging and never leaving.

SOCIAL AND PERSONAL FACTORS THAT INFLUENCE A POSITIVE OUTCOME OF CULTURE SHOCK

Learning to Trust the New Environment

In this section I identify social and personal factors that helped me trust the new environment. Salient interactional variables proved to consist of neighborliness, showing respect, making an impact on the host society, and again, having options. Personal factors include egregiousness, tolerance of danger, transportable support system, and love of self-actualization.

Neighborliness

Natives of North Louisiana pride themselves on being helpful to their neighbors. Our neighbors mowed the lawn, offered the use of the telephone, and watered the houseplants when we were away. Offered pay, the teenager next door was insulted. His response was, "why shoot, that's just bein' a good neighbor, isn't it?" (California teenagers work for pay, period.) In the work setting, certain special colleagues led me by the hand, helped me fill out forms, and took me to lunch. Other colleagues made a point of seeing that the emigrants had invitations to holiday dinners.

Showing Respect

This variable is exemplified by attentive listening. One expects ideological conficts, but the emigrant wants and needs to have her or his foreign ideas considered thoughtfully. For example, most students showed respect by listening attentively, and responding favorably. Generally, fellow faculty members treated me with tolerance. However, certain of my educational strategies, radical by Shreveport standards, were rejected outright by some of my colleagues. As Thompson (1982) put it, the shovel hit the stone. They would not even compromise. I almost folded my tent right then and there. But when all else failed, we did a study about it (Harris, Stern, & Woodard, 1982).

Making an Impact on the Host Society

This variable ties closely with showing respect. Having listened with care, does the host act on at least some suggestions? I am convinced that this factor is vital to the preservation of the emigrant's self-esteem, sense of safety, and hence, successful resolution of shock. The most exciting event of my $2\frac{1}{2}$ years in North Louisiana was the production of creative works: students and faculty published and presented papers at national meetings. The south has long been known as an area from which, for one reason or another, few nursing publications emerge. My perception of the situation led me to the belief that I influenced the increased productivity.

Having Options

I consider myself fortunate indeed that I live in a time when having a little education, and being in a popular profession allows one almost unlimited options. I also have the great good fortune of having a mate who is supportive, stimulating, and *mobile*. If being stuck in a foreign culture were added to the other variables in culture shock, the trauma might seem unbearable.

Personal Factors in the Successful Resolution of Culture Shock

Turning one's life upside down is not for everyone. From my experience, and from the observation of other shock breakers, I suggest that the following personal characteristics contribute to successful resolution of culture shock.

Egregiousness

One of the characteristics that seems important in successful transplantation is a certain willingness to stand out in a crowd. A willingness to stand out allows one to maintain a certain integrity of ideology, yet withstand the discomfort of not being one-of-the-gang. An example from my data illustrates this point. When describing my position in a foreign area to a visitor from California, I said, "It's kind of fun being considered an exotic," to which the visitor replied, "but Phyllis, you always have been."

Danger Tolerance

Closely akin to egregiousness is a willingness to be a risk taker and a thrill seeker. Kelsey (1979) tells us that in the transfer of telephone company employees, only persons willing to "risk" the move should be asked to do so. Without these qualities, relocation might be tolerated poorly.

Transportable Support System

Lin, Tazuma, and Masuda (1979), writing about Vietnamese refugees in Seattle cited marital status and family groupings as important factors in adapting to the host country. I would add that the option of telephoning old friends back home helps one tolerate the transition period. Having networks or connection within one's profession, church, or culture is another important variable.

Love of Self-Actualization

As a native Californian, I am "into" self-actualization. According to Maslow (1954), I can afford this pursuit because all my other needs for survival have been met. Self-actualization receives the lowest priority when compared to a need for food and shelter, for example. I can think of no better process for self-learning, that is, self-actualization, than relocation. How better to see-yourself-as-others-see-you than to become a foreigner—with an accent, yet! Stouffer's (1955/1966) claim that culture shock provides a learning experience for developing great tolerance and appreciation of the strange and different holds true for me.

IMPLICATIONS FOR TRANSCULTURAL NURSING

Nursing Shock

One of my strategies for getting through the day during a crisis situation is to build a cognitive map constructed of the strands of previous and similar situations. Having moved frequently from job to job as many nurses do, I had prior knowledge of that experience. Thus I was able to say, "oh yes, I remember, it takes 2 months to operationalize a new job."

Aamodt (1978), writing about culture shock tells us, "in transfers from one hospital unit to another, one job to another, one health worker to another, the phenomenon can be experienced by patients, health workers, and researchers alike" (p. 9). I suggest that the situation of nurses or teachers moving from one position to another may be commonplace, but it is nonetheless traumatic, confusing, and could be ameliorated with certain supports. One quite simple yet effective strategy would be acknowledgement of shock by members of the host culture. In Shreveport, I kept saying, "I'm in culture shock, I am not functioning normally." But it was weeks to months before I was heard. Finally, as I began to emerge, my colleagues said, "oh yes, I see, you *were* in shock, weren't you?"

The 2-week orientation period (if indeed that exists) proves quite insufficient for the new employee. I could not even *hear* anything the first 2 weeks. Orientation ideally might go on for a year or more. New medical residents often receive one month's orientation to a service, plus a year's guided practice. To my knowledge, no nursing program, health institution, or university offers support of this kind to employees.

Patient Shock

Orientation for patients is almost nonexistent in today's health care settings. If the patient is oriented at all, it comes during her or his introduction to the facility when she or he cannot hear due to the high anxiety state of most newly admitted patients. As has been previously noted, it is well to remember that no amount of prior teaching softens culture shock. Ramsden (1980), suggests that being incarcerated in a hospital is very much like becoming a prisoner. We may need to learn language that transcends the lay and health culture. And as Ramsden suggests, "the technical language of the staff is difficult to understand and often sounds portentous, if not calamitous" (p. 290).

CONCLUSIONS

Culture shock offers the same potential for growth that any crisis affords; in other words, with pain can come profit. When the familiar frames of reference dissolve, the possibility occurs for observing new vistas, often those of greater clarity and depth. The opportunity for developing new and unexpected sources of support should not be minimized. One also has the chance of trying out new behaviors, some of which may prove to be more adaptive than former ways of interacting. I learned, for example, to behave toward physicians as colleagues, rather than as *the enemy,* and with splendid results! I realize this marks me as a heretic, but as Rodgers (1981) tells us, this kind of nurse-physician relationship is necessary if our profession of nursing is to emerge from its adolescence.

Crisis theory teaches us that with the right kinds of support, persons can recover from disaster at a higher level of functioning. If we can learn to provide support for the victim of culture shock, whether immigrant, emigrant, nurse, teacher, or patient, the same kind of improved quality of life may occur. Without support, less desirable outcomes of ghettoism and prolonged cultural identity crisis may result.

REFERENCES

Aamodt, A. M. (1978). Culture. In A. L. Clark (Ed.), *Culture childbearing health professionals.* Philadelphia: Davis.

Beiser, M., & Collomb, H. (1981). Mastering change: Epidemiological and case studies in Senegal, West Africa. *American Journal of Psychiatry, 65,* 1352.

Brein, M., & David, K. H. (1971). Intercultural communication and the adjustment of the sojourner. *Psychology Bulletin, 76,* 212–230.

Brink, P. J., & Saunders, J. M. (1976). Cultural shock: Theoretical and applied. In P. J. Brink (Ed.), *Transcultural nursing.* Englewood Cliffs: Prentice-Hall.

Durkheim, E. (1915). *The elementary forms of the religious life.* New York: Free Press.

Durkheim, E. (1930). *Rules of sociological methods.* Paris: Alcan.

Durkheim, E. (1947). *Division of labor in society.* Glencoe, IL: Free Press.

Feinberg, R. (1979). Schneider's symbolic culture theory: An appraisal. *Current Anthropology. 20,* 541–560.

Glaser, B., & Strauss, A. (1967). *The discovery of grounded theory.* Chicago: Aldine.

Glittenberg, J. E. (1981). An ethnographic approach to the problem of health assessment and program planning: Project Genesis. In P. Morley (Ed.), *Published Proceedings of the Sixth National Transcultural Nursing Conference,* (pp. 143–153). Salt Lake City: University of Utah Press.

Harris, C. C., Stern, P. N., & Woodward, E. (1982). *Summative evaluation of masters students in nursing: A national survey.* Unpublished manuscript.

Kelsey, J. E. (1979). The stress of relocation: Helping employees ease the pain. *Occupational Health and Safety, January–February,* 26–30.

Lin, M. K., Tazuma, L., & Masuda, M. (1979). Adaptational problems of Vietnamese refugees. *Archives of General Psychiatry, 36,* 955–961.

Lundstedt, S. (1963). An introduction to some evolving problems in cross-cultural research. *Journal of Social Issues, July,* 1–9.

Maslow, A. H. (1954). *Motivation and personality.* New York: Harper.

Oberg, K. (1954). *Culture shock.* Indianapolis: Bobbs-Merrill.

Olien, M. D. (1978). *The human myth.* New York: Harper & Row.

Ramsden, E. L. (1980). Values in conflict: Hospital culture shock. *Physical Therapy, 60,* 289–292.

Rodgers, J. A. (1981). Toward professional adulthood. *Nursing Outlook, 28,* 478–481.

Stern, P. N. (1982). A comparison of culturally approved behaviors and beliefs between Pilipina-American immigrant women, American-born dominant culture women and Western female nurses: Religiosity of health care. In P. Morley (Ed.), *Proceedings of the Sixth Annual Transcultural Nursing Conference.* Salt Lake City: Transcultural Nursing Society, 85–95.

Stern, P. N. (1980). Grounded theory methodology: Its uses and processes. *Image, 12,* 20–23.

Stouffer, S. A. (1966). *Communism, conformity and civil liberties.* New York: Doubleday. (Originally published 1955)

Taft, R. (1976). Coping with unfamiliar cultures. In N. Warren (Ed.), *Studies in cross-cultural psychology* (Vol. 1).

Thompson, J. L. (1982, September). *Synchronic paradigm development and mystification in transcultural nursing research: The case of Indochinese refugees.* Paper presented at the Seventh Annual Transcultural Nursing Conference, Seattle, Washington.

Toffler, A. (1970). *Future shock.* New York: Random House.

Tylor, E. B. (1958). *Primitive culture* (2 vols.). New York: Harper & Row, Harper Torchbooks. (Originally published 1871)

WOMEN'S HEALTH AND THE SELF–CARE PARADOX:
A MODEL TO GUIDE SELF–CARE READINESS

Phyllis Noerager Stern, DNS, RN, FAAN
Dalhousie University School of Nursing, Halifax, Nova Scotia

Chandice C. Harris, MSN, RN
University of Michigan School of Nursing, Ann Arbor

Based on the teaching of their culture, women have reasons for their health practices. Nurses, in turn, based on the teaching of their culture of origin, with superimposed professional "scientific" culture beliefs, have reasons for the health behaviors they think their clients should practice. We call these beliefs *cultural reasoning.* When they clash, culture shock occurs, possibly leading to power struggles, fencing, and withdrawal from care, or the giving of care.

We describe a model consisting of four self-care paradigms: two congruent and two noncongruent. Understanding them can help the nurse assess the client's and the nurse's self-care readiness.

North Americans schooled in a social world that reinforces independent thought and action would seem to be logical proponents of self-care ideologies. It is therefore understandable that self-care nursing models such as Orem's (1971) are widely accepted in our profession. How appropriate it seems for North American nurses to encourage North American clients to manage their own care and thereby develop more independence. A stated belief in the idea of self-care implies no real readiness for it however, for either the nurse or the client. Self-care is the professional nurses' published ideology, not necessarily the model in practice. The client may never have heard of it. By this we mean that the nurse may be unwilling to surrender professional control or be intimidated by the control exerted by the medical model. The client may not understand what self-care is all about, why the nurse values it, or what its value might be.

In a qualitative meta-analysis of seven nursing studies, we discovered a variable that we call the *self-care paradox.* The paradox exists when an interaction between client and nurse is complicated by a number of processes within certain contexts. The resulting cognitive dissonance prevents facilitation of the process. As nurse and client meet, each employs what we call separate *cultural reasoning* within their separate cultural context, about the client's expressed health care need. Not understanding one another's cultural prescriptions and proscriptions, they experience culture shock. Culture shock is manifested by fencing, power struggles, and withdrawal. The processes are further complicated within a context of interdependent practice. These contexts and processes are seen to occur within four self-care paradigms, two congruent and two noncongruent.

Cultural elasticity and showing respect are two variables that tend to bridge lay and professional cultural points of view, allowing self-care processes to continue. These two transcending variables seem to be enhanced when they occur within the context of independent nursing practice.

Our description of these variables, contexts, and paradigms provide a guide to self-care readiness that the nurse may use in practice. We define the variable self-care generically in order to encompass the conceptual intent of taking-care-of-self rather than as a construct formed from a single nursing model. We used the American Nurses Association 1980 Social Policy Statement to define nursing as "... the diagnosis and treatment of human responses to actual or potential health problems."

QUALITATIVE META-ANALYSIS

We traced the variable self-care through the data and findings from seven qualitative nursing studies. We used grounded theory techniques (Glaser & Strauss, 1967; Glaser, 1978; Stern, 1980; Stern, Allen, & Moxley, 1982) to discover the limits, dimensions, properties, and contexts of the variable, prominent in all seven studies. In this way a qualitative *meta-analysis* was done. Webster defines the word *meta* as "later, more highly organized or specialized (in) form ... more comprehensive: transcending" (Woolf, 1977, p. 721). O'Flynn (1982) described computer techniques of meta-analysis as "... using old data to answer new questions ... the integration of findings, the analysis of analyses ..." (p. 314). O'Flynn warns that "Meta-analysts lack the first hand experience of the primary research team. Therefore, researchers may not have an adequate grasp of the actual treatment or program under investigation." (p. 316).

Both investigators in this study (Stern & Harris, 1983) were involved with all of the seven nursing studies mentioned above. Therefore, there was no problem of unfamiliarity with the original data. Findings from the following studies were used as data for the meta-analysis: Brocato's (1982) study of pain assessment on an orthopedic ward, Moore's (1982) research on menopausal women, Scott's (1982) study of the childbearing beliefs of northern Louisiana black persons, Harris' (1982) study of cultural decision-making involved in circumcision, Stern's work on culture shock (Stern & Cousins, 1982), Stern and Harris' case study of a high-risk maternity patient (1983), and Stern's study on childbearing beliefs of Filipino immigrants (Stern, 1981). Additional data and help with the analysis came from nursing educators, students, and practitioners in Louisiana and Nova Scotia (Stern, 1982a); the Philippine Islands (Stern, 1982b); and a Nursing Conference in Madrid (Stern, 1983). The mixed, lay and professional study population of about 500 persons, represents Caucasian, Black, Filipino, and other Asian groups.

FINDINGS

Meta-analysis of the seven studies indicates that enculturating experiences differ both between and among lay and professional groups. Depending on age, curriculum exposures, and to some degree, cultural subgroup, clients and nurses had beliefs that either favored self-care, or found it undesirable. The two groups often had different conceptions of what "taking-care-of-self" meant. Furthermore, lay and professional cultures were generally ignorant concerning how the other group defined self-care. This was more than a linguistic problem in which clients simply lacked knowledge of professional terminology. The problem seemed to be more profound in that the separate groups had insufficient information and sensitivity to be able to understand the point of view of the other.

We discovered four paradigms that define self-care perspectives between nurse and client, two congruent and two incongruent. Figure 1 shows that in paradigm 1 both nurse and client agree on the value of self-care. In paradigm 2, the client values self-care while the nurse does not. In paradigm 3, the nurse values self-care but the client does not, and in paradigm 4, both client and nurse agree that self-care is undesirable. Interactional processes are consistent throughout the paradigms.

Paradigm 1: Teamwork?

A contextual congruency wherein nurse and client agree that an optimal health state can best be achieved and/or maintained when the client practices self-care would seem to offer ideal conditions for nurse and client to become working partners of the health team. As Woolery states, "A key concept for the nurse to grasp is that man, as

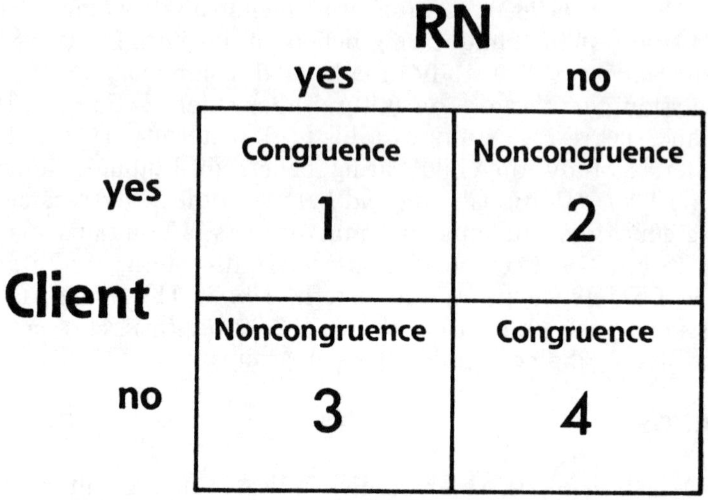

RN

	yes	no

	yes	Congruence **1**	Noncongruence **2**
Client			
	no	Noncongruence **3**	Congruence **4**

Figure 1. A model to guide self-care readiness.

a self-care agent, is capable of making decisions and working towards goals with deliberate action." (p. 33). We questioned the use of teamwork since our data indicate that although nurse and client sometimes work as a team, because of their cultural inflexibility, nurses and clients tend to set separate self-care goals. Each believes she or he knows perfectly well what is best for the client, based on her or his own cultural reasoning.

The example we use to illustrate the teamwork paradigm is normal pregnancy. Pregnancy, generally a healthy physical state, lends itself quite well to notions of self-management of care. The nurse acts as advisor and monitor of the physical state, and as a source of information and support. The healthy pregnant woman can learn about self-care practices through books, TV, prenatal classes and by consulting her family. Problems may arise when the client or nurse or both have cultural beliefs that the other either knows nothing of or fails to understand.

The interactional pattern that ensues seems fairly consistent. When nurse and client encounter what they consider inexplicable behavior on the part of the other they are both thrown into the cognitive dissonance of culture shock. They struggle for power, fence off their territories, and withdraw. For example, a pregnant woman may follow her mother's advice about eating certain foods, but avoid telling the nurse the true content of her diet. A frustrated nurse, on the other hand, rather than argue with a recalcitrant patient may avoid the issue or the patient. Figure 2 depicts these processes. The dynamics of paradigm 1 are described in more detail in the case study that follows in the next chapter.

Paradigm 2: Troublemaker

When the client has firm ideas about self-care, but the nurse has a "we-know-best" attitude, the same processes occur as do in paradigm 1. In this paradigm, after culture shock occurs accompanied by fencing and withdrawal, the client is labeled a troublemaker and neither client nor nurse can understand why the other is "acting that way." We found particularly vivid examples of this sort of interaction in Brocato's (1982) pain study, where nurses often thought they could use objective means, like time interval, to measure the subjective experience of a patient's pain.

According to our data, a patient with a painful injury might become aware that the prescribed analgesic dose of medication would be ineffective in 2 hours, and that to wait the regulation 4 hours for more medication would mean that the medication would never overcome the pain. Often this patient knew from past experience that her or his body was particularly resistant to the effects of analgesics. Nevertheless, in this study, patients' pleas for more frequent medication were not well understood by many nurses. Nurses tended to interpret the patients' request as an indication of drug dependency. The patient who insisted on medication at nonprescribed hours was called "troublemaker" or "crock,"

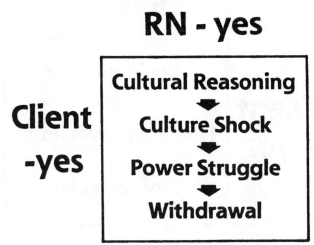

Figure 2. Paradigm 1: Teamwork?

by some nurses. The troublemaker paradigm processes can be seen in Figure 3.

Paradigm 3: Noncompliance

When the nurse sees the client as self-care "agency" (Orem, 1971, p. 13), but the client sees the nurse as someone to "take care of me," we have both a conceptual and an educational incongruency (Stewart, Lambie, Downe-Wamboldt, & Slater, 1983). In this paradigm, following culture shock, fencing, and withdrawal, the patient is either considered "lazy," or "noncompliant." The example we use to illustrate this paradigm is that of Filipino immigrants. Filipino women raised in the Philippines are taught that part of taking care of themselves after giving birth is to submit to bed rest and total nursing care. The nurse who reacts in an indifferent manner is seen by these women as someone who does not like them. Other clients as well, who are unschooled in self-care ideologies, often see this nurse as lazy because she does not provide them with "service." The processes in paradigm 3 are illustrated in Figure 4.

Paradigm 4: Forced Dependence

When nurse and client agree that self-care is inadvisable they fall into paradigm 4. The crisis victim in panic belongs in this cell, as

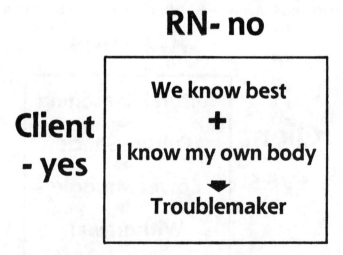

Figure 3. Paradigm 2: Troublemaker.

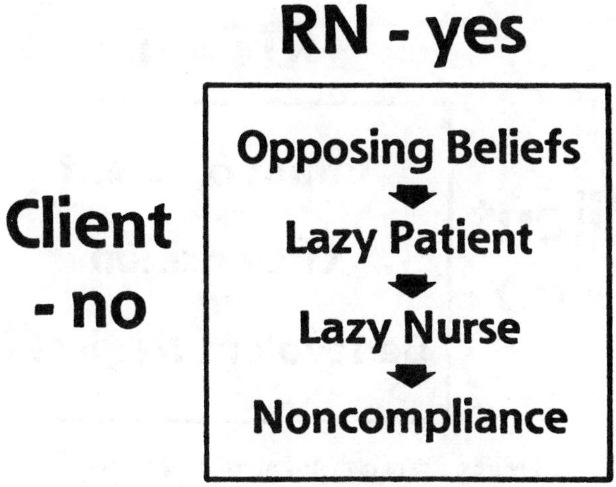

RN - yes

Client
- no

Opposing Beliefs
⬇
Lazy Patient
⬇
Lazy Nurse
⬇
Noncompliance

Figure 4. Paradigm 3: Noncompliance.

well as the woman in second stage labor. However, we exclude the unconscious patient, since all the other cells represent an element of choice for both client and nurse ("Graduate Students," 1982). The example we chose from the data that shows a possible choice, concerns parents of a newborn boy and the issue of circumcision because "parents become self-care agents for their infants and children" (Woolery, 1983, p. 33). Since 1975, the American Academy of Pediatrics has maintained that routine circumcision of the newborn is unnecessary. Therefore, a decision about whether or not to circumcise a baby boy is based on the cultural prescriptions of the parents, and to some extent, the nurse (Harris, 1982). The nurse who believes that self-care is inadvisable will either neglect to advise the parents of their options concerning circumcision or neglect the parents' cultural beliefs in the matter and force the issue with an outpouring of nursing beliefs. The passive parents in this case take the nurse's prescription on faith. By contrast, the nurse *proponent* of self-care (cell one, *teamwork*) might practice benevolent neglect in two ways. If she determines that the parents' cultural belief in circumcision is strong, she can simply avoid negative references to circumcision. On the other hand, if the nurse determines the parents' cultural opposition to circumcision to be firm, the nurse can become client advocate, helping to see that the baby's foreskin is benignly neglected. If, however, the nurse fails to take the cultural part of the other, the same processes occur in this paradigm that occur in the other three. Figure 5 illustrates paradigm 4.

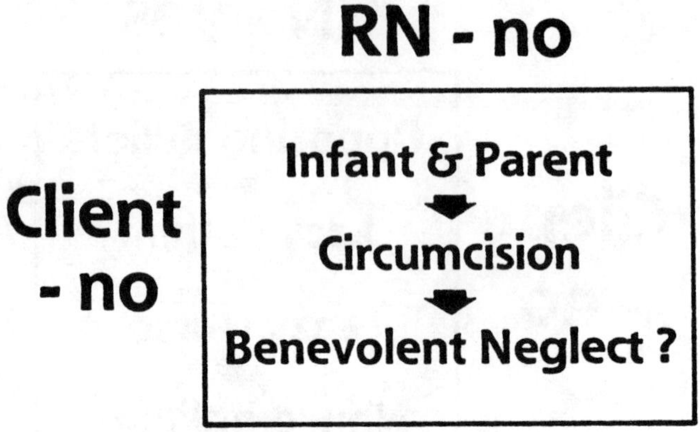

RN - no

Client - no

Infant & Parent
⬇
Circumcision
⬇
Benevolent Neglect ?

Figure 5. Paradigm 4: Forced dependency.

EXTENSIONS AND LIMITATIONS OF THE PARADIGMS

If we consider the paradigm dynamics as existing in their purest form at the point furthest from the neighboring cells and more defused toward their common borders, we can see that in paradigm 1 client and nurse may work as a team. When the client, however, exercises more self-care options than the nurse is comfortable with, they may move into the second paradigm. As the client asserts her or his right to follow her or his lay cultural judgment, the nurse may consider the client a troublemaker, unwilling to follow sound advice. By contrast, if the client decides that open confrontation is not working, or is not a comfortable style, the client uses passive-aggressive strategies in order to follow her particular cultural reasoning. Such strategies as telling the nurse, "I forgot to take the medication." or "I had a big dinner last night and that's why my weight is up" are examples from our data. This client tends to be labeled noncompliant as shown in paradigm 3.

In paradigm 3 we find, on the one hand, the noncompliant Filipino acting on her own cultural reasoning about self-care (that is, anti-self-care in actuality). As we move toward paradigm 4, we find, for example, the alcoholic, who says, and who seems to believe, "Nurse, I just can't do it." The nurse insists, "It's up to you to stay dry," but in this case, the nurse is asking the client to do something that the client feels unable to do.

The closer clients move toward cell four, the more often they ask the nurse for direction and the more they seem unable to manage self-care. We suggest that paradigm 4 is dynamic in nature and seems to describe the patient in acute crisis. As the panic of crisis narrows the perceptual field and diminishes the ability to concentrate, the client may be unable to complete simple tasks, read a form, or understand directions. At this point, both nurse and client agree that self-care is out of the question until the panic subsides.

Comparison of Paradigms 2 and 3

At first glance, paradigms 2 and 3 seem to be reverse mirror images of one another. On closer inspection we find a dramatic difference in the role played by the nurse vis-à-vis the general North American cultural view of her role. That is to say that the stereotypical nurse is one who administers care, and that care involves doing things for people. The view of the nurse as one who helps the client find her or his way to self-management of care has not found its way into the general cultural picture of the nurse role. Therefore, the nurse who puts self-care ideologies into practice runs contrary to general cultural beliefs—always an uneasy position in which to find oneself. For this reason, paradigm 2, the troublemaker sequence, tends to be a stable one. As the client becomes more active, demanding control over body or mind, the nurse in turn becomes more active in her attempts to control this independent behavior. The reasons for this become clear when we consider that even though the nurse may have learned self-care principles in school or from reading nursing literature, the nurse's deep-seated norm for the nurse role is as one who administers care and controls. If the client seems to the nurse to be resisting control, a safer strategy, it seems, would be for the nurse to do something rather than nothing. Many nurses perceive that society holds them responsible for the client's well-being. Therefore it seems more familiar, and safer for the nurse to stay on top of things. The client who is always "one down" to the nurse's "one-up" position, feels powerless to change the system. Therefore, the client in paradigm 2 usually leaves the care situation vowing never to return.

Paradigm 3 holds out more hope. Since the nurse learned an ideology foreign to her previous cultural norms, it seems plausible to expect that the client too would be capable of learning these self-care ideologies. Learning is the key here. To expect a client to become more active in the management of care while the nurse assumes a more passive role requires that the nurse engage in a comprehensive educational program to explain the value for the client of self-care. Because nurses often neglect this educational step, they become frustrated by client noncompliance.

The mistake most nurses in our study made was that they assumed their clients knew what they were talking about. This brings us full circle back to cultural reasoning. Cultural reasoning carries with it contributing variables of cultural deafness and cultural blindness. Neither client nor nurse can hear one another because the words they use have different symbolic meanings, and each misses verbal clues given by the other because of their own cultural centeredness. Our data show that nurse and client persistence can resolve these problems. However, the client who leaves the care situation prior to resolution of these problems feels diminished and discouraged by her experience.

The interrupting variables described in the paradigms above are more likely to occur or be reinforced within the context of interdependent practice or nursing action, and are less likely to occur within independent practice situations. This concept is further illustrated in the case study that follows.

TRANSCENDING VARIABLES

We discovered in our data that even when lay and health cultures have differing perceptions about self-care, the variables of *cultural elasticity,* and *showing respect* help to overcome interruptions in the self-care nursing process seen in the four paradigms. By cultural elasticity, we mean an ability to understand the cultural prescriptions and proscriptions of the other. Some nurses and clients gain cultural elasticity through experience and knowledge. Cultural elasticity represents the wisdom gained from the politics of making the system work. Nurses or clients who gain cultural elasticity learn to operate within the cultural prescriptions of the other.

Data from the seven studies indicate that showing respect aids cooperative interaction between client and nurse. While persons involved still experience the culture shock that comes with cultural reasoning, treating one another with respect helps to facilitate interaction in spite of a lack of understanding. We noted with interest that both client and nurse seem to require a show of respect from the other.

The two transcending variables were more likely to occur when the nurse's practice was independent (Dickson & Lee-Villasenor, 1982), meaning in the presence of defined *nursing* action, as opposed to care involving doctor's orders, lab results, and the like. Intervening variables, such as doctor's orders and lab results, tend to vitiate the judgment of the nurse.

USING THE GUIDE IN PRACTICE

The paradigms described here can be used to test self-care in practice (Hutchinson, 1982; Faucett, 1983). Consulting the four cells of the model, the nurse has at hand a guide to assess the client's readiness for self-care and the nurse's own readiness as well. Cells one and four, the *teamwork* and *forced dependency* cells, depict fairly clear cut entities; teamwork representing the ideal, and forced dependency, a second-choice situation. Cells two and three give us a guide for considering our options.

In cell two, the *troublemaker* cell, where the client and nurse struggle for control of care, we believe it is incumbent upon the nurse to examine the client's reasons for demanding control. Nursing diagnoses such as, "acting out behavior, response to crisis, drug dependency, or self-destructiveness," may or may not be appropriate. More often than not, such diagnoses serve to cloud the issue, and may well be the result of the nurse's cultural deafness and blindness. Considered within the framework of the self-care paradox model, the clash between the client and nurse may be the result of the nurse's misinterpretation of the client's cultural reasoning about self-care. To return to the pain study illustration once more, our data show that some enlightened nurses perceived that the patient with atypical demands for pain medication quite simply requires alteration in medication regime. Two statements made by nurses stay with us: "Where pain is concerned, you have to be willing to suspend disbelief," and "After 40 years in this business, I have learned something very simple. If the patient says she hurts, I believe her—works real well."

In other instances it seems the nurse must examine her own motives for insisting on control. Does the need to be in command belong to the patient or the nurse?

Cell three, the *noncompliant* paradigm, gives the nurse equal opportunity for examining her practice. What is the reason behind the client's noncompliance? Why is it that the client seems unwilling to do what the nurse asks? Does the client's cultural reasoning forbid following the nurse's prescription? Does the client have a cultural prescription that supercedes the nurse's prescription? We may not appreciate the health rituals required by cultures other than our own. Indeed, for ethnic groups that look, talk, and act like we do, we may forget the separation and therefore the differences between professional and lay cultures.

When the nurse feels ready to assume the more passive role of client-managed care, but the client seems unwilling or unready, we believe the nurse can better assess the situation by thinking about the nurse-client interaction in terms of cultural reasoning. We believe these cases may call for consultation with a nurse anthropologist, sociologist, or other nurse scientist.

The transition period between nurse-directed care and client-directed care may be slowed because of the client's belief system, because the client does not value self-care, or because the client simply is not ready for it, as in the case of the not-dry-yet alcoholic.

In sum, our self-care paradox model can be seen in the following abbreviated ways:

1. Teamwork: the ideal.
2. Troublemaker: who insists on control and why?
3. Noncompliant: is the transition slowed because of values or dependency?
4. Forced dependency: little or no option for now.

CONCLUSION

Meta-analysis of seven nursing studies indicates that self-care nursing processes become interrupted or enhanced on the basis of the symbolic meaning and values of client and nurse and the way these are interpreted during the nurse-client interaction. We conclude that an understanding of the client's expression of need seems beyond the range of vision of all but the most experienced, knowledgeable, and wise nurses.

REFERENCES

American Nurses' Association (1980). *Nursing a social policy statement.* Kansas: Author. (NP-63 35M)

Brocato, C. (1982). *Right and left brain nursing: Pain assessment on an orthopedic ward.* Unpublished Master's thesis, Northwestern State University of Louisiana, College of Nursing, Shreveport, Louisiana.

Dickson, G. L., & Lee-Villasenor, H. (1982). Nursing theory and practice: A self-care approach. *Advances in Nursing Science. October,* 29–40.

Fawcett, J. (1983). *Research seminar.* Sigma Theta Tau Clinical Nursing Study Tour, Marbella, Spain, July 18.

Glaser, B. G. (1978). *Theoretical sensitivity.* Mill Valley, CA: Sociology Press.

Glaser, B., & Strauss, A. (1967). *The discovery of grounded theory.* Chicago: Aldine.

Graduate students seminar in nursing theories (1982). Northwestern State University, College of Nursing, Shreveport, Louisiana, September 16.

Harris, C. C. (1982). Circumcision: A cultural decision. In C. N. Uhl & J. Uhl

(Eds.) *Proceedings of the Seventh Annual Transcultural Nursing Conference.* Salt Lake City: University of Utah Press.

Hutchinson, S. A. (1983). *Research seminar.* Sigma Theta Tau Clinical Nursing Study Tour, Seville, Spain, July 9.

Moore, P. G. (1982). *Response to menopause of selected northern Louisiana women.* Unpublished Master's Thesis. Northwestern State University of Louisiana, College of Nursing, Shreveport, Louisiana.

O'Flynn, A. J. (1982). Meta-analysis. *Nursing Research, 31*(5), 314–316.

Orem, D. E. (1971). *Nursing: Concepts of practice.* St. Louis: McGraw-Hill.

Scott, M. D. S. (1982). *Childbearing beliefs of northern Louisiana blacks.* Unpublished Master's thesis. Northwestern State University of Louisiana, College of Nursing, Shreveport, Louisiana.

Stern, P. N. (1980). Grounded theory methodology: Its uses and processes. *Image, 12*(1), 20–23.

Stern, P. N. (1981). Solving problems of cross-cultural health teaching: The Filipino childbearing family. *Image, 13*(2), 47–50.

Stern, P. N. (1982a). *The nurse as research instrument.* Research and Development Series, Killam Library, Dalhousie University, Halifax, Nova Scotia, October 25.

Stern, P. N. (1982b). Nursing education in the United States: The emergence of transcultural nursing research. School of Nursing, University of the Philippines, Manila, December 9.

Stern, P. N. (1983). *Perceptual differences in self-care between nurse and client: Issues of culture shock and control.* Madrid Nursing Research Conference, co-sponsored by Universidad Compluense and Sigma Theta Tau, July 8–9.

Stern, P. N., Allen, L. M., & Moxley, P. A. (1982). The nurse as grounded theorist: History, process, and uses. *Review Journal of Philosophy and Social Science, 7*(1, 2), 200–215.

Stern, P. N., & Cousins, M. E. B. (1982). Culture shock as a positive force: Surviving West Coast to northern Louisiana relocation. In C. N. Uhl & J. Uhl (Eds.), *Published Proceedings of the Seventh Annual Transcultural Nursing Conference.* Salt Lake City: University of Utah.

Stern, P. N., & Harris, C. C. (1983). Self-care from the patient's perspective: Issues of culture shock and control. Theoretical analysis and case study. Meta-analysis research. Unpublished research report.

Stewart, M. J., Lambie, E., Downe-Wamboldt, B., & Slater, M. (1983). *Overcoming barriers to implementing primary health care.* A brief to the Select Committee on Health of the Provincial Government of Nova Scotia, from the School of Nursing, Dalhousie University, Halifax, Nova Scotia, January 12.

Woolery, L. F. (1983). Self-care for the obstetrical patient. *Journal of Obstetric, Gynecologic, and Neonatal Nursing, 12,* 33–38.

Woolf, H. B. (Ed.). (1977). *Webster's New Collegiate Dictionary.* Springfield, MA: Merriam.

WOMEN'S HEALTH AND THE SELF–CARE PARADOX: CASE STUDY AND ANALYSIS

Chandice C. Harris, MSN, RN
University of Michigan School of Nursing, Ann Arbor

Phyllis Noerager Stern, DNS, RN, FAAN
Dalhousie University School of Nursing, Halifax, Nova Scotia

A case study analysis is used to demonstrate the theory of the self-care paradox. This case involves a client who is also a health care professional and her experience with a high risk pregnancy. The professional caregivers and the client differed in their perception of the appropriate self-care agency when the pregnancy became problematic. The key components of the paradox are highlighted as the actors progress through interpersonal and intraprofessional negotiations and realignments of roles. An adaptive self-care approach then evolves. From the meta-analysis of previous studies and the case study a predictive model for self-care readiness is developed.

The practice of self-care seems especially appropriate during the experience of normal pregnancy. Prenatal care, nutrition, exercise, and childbirth education are all areas over which the client can maintain a measure of control, choice, and power (Woolery, 1983; Dickson & Lee-Villasenor, 1982). During a high-risk pregnancy, however, loss of control, choice, and power predictably occur in direct response to the danger of the risk, and the need for the latest technology to alleviate the risk. Self-care practice then becomes more challenging for both the patient to maintain and the caregiver to allow.

Through a case study analysis of a high-risk pregnancy, we examine the variable *self-care paradox* from the client's perspective. Paradox refers to a conflict between what is espoused by care-givers and clients, and what in reality occurs in regard to the practice of self-care. In this case study, discrepancies between theory and practice lead the well intentioned care-giver and the conscientious client to experience a relationship fraught with cultural *reasoning, culture shock, fencing,* and *power struggles,* resulting in tangled lines of responsibility for self-care. Awareness and valuing of the processes of *cultural elasticity* and *showing respect* transcended the paradox of self-care practice difficulties, and in this way, clear lines of responsibility were established and a quality pregnancy outcome ensued.

METHOD

The method we used to analyze the data was twofold, the present case study having been the initial emphasis. The factors that influenced care in this case puzzled and disturbed us. With this case as the irritant, we began tracing the variable self-care through six other nursing studies that we had been involved with (Brocato, 1982; Harris, 1982; Moore, 1982; Scott, 1982). We conducted a qualitative meta-analysis (or analysis of analyses) from a data bank that included material from approximately 500 persons.

Our analysis of the data was based on the grounded theory method described by Glaser and Strauss (1967; Glaser, 1978; Stern, 1980; Stern, Allen, & Moxley, 1982). We used both the findings and the data from the previous studies and the present case to form our theory, self-care paradox.

Case Study Method

The case study research method has recently met with renewed endorsements. Once criticized as worthless to the establishment of nursing as a science, the case study approach has gained recognition as a method responsive to building a descriptive base for nursing research (Stern, Allen, & Moxley, 1982; Barnard, 1983). In fact, a national call requests that nurses report case studies that identify the "it" of nursing (Barnard, 1983). In this manner, the practice of nursing and the research of nursing combine to reveal the phenomenon of nursing (Dickson & Lee-Villasenor, 1982).

Case Study Report

Carrie, a 29-year-old Caucasian, married mother of two, and a maternal clinical nurse specialist discovered to her and her 35-year-old husband's surprise and shock that she was pregnant. Previous infertility problems had made pregnancy seem remote, though the couple nevertheless practiced birth control. However, their method of pregnancy prevention obviously failed.

Carrie, who had a high-risk pregnancy history, immediately sought care from an obstetrician (OB) who was just beginning practice, having recently completed a specialty residency. In addition, during the first trimester, she contracted with two certified nurse midwives (CNM) to handle the normal aspects of pregnancy, labor, and delivery, while the obstetrician agreed to provide medical back-up if necessary. All members of this health care team (CNM, physician, patient), espoused self-care theory beliefs. It is important to note that the physician, even though he had worked with the CNMs in the public health sector, had never shared the care of a private patient with them. He voiced concerns about his role and responsibility for client management during the pregnancy, birth, and postpartum period. There were other firsts in this case. The two midwives had managed the care for private patients along with their work in the public hospital, but this was their first case of client management in partnership with a private physician. Carrie, a professional colleague of all three of her caregivers, had placed herself under the care of midwives for the first time. For all four of these persons some aspects of their anticipated roles were new and untried.

Another important part of this case study was taken on by Ann, Carrie's faculty colleague. Ann's assigned role was that of friend, her assumed role became that of nurse.

Due to Carrie's past history, a serum glucose screen and ultrasound were completed during the second trimester and proved normal. Then, early into the last trimester, Carrie began showing urinary ketosis. Ketosis occurs when the body uses fat for energy instead of glucose. It is one of the signs that may indicate pregnancy-induced diabetes.

The CNM suggested that Carrie monitor her urinary output for ketones at home and report findings to the health care team. The physician, when informed, seemed unimpressed with the data. In fact, his suggestion was to, "stop checking your urine."

Symptoms increased. After two weeks of ketosis, weight loss, glysuria (glucose in the urine), labile hypertension, dizziness, tachycardia following meals, and shakiness prior to meals, another glucose screen and a 2,000 calorie high-protein diet was ordered. Even though the glucose screen was high normal, symptoms persisted. Carrie requested that her physician order a full glucose tolerance test (GTT). He refused, stating that the effects of ketosis on the fetus, namely anoxia, was "theoretical."

While sympathetic, the CNMs adopted a "wait and see attitude" explaining that the symptoms might be transient. Meanwhile, Carrie sought advice from her colleague, Ann, also a maternal child clinical nurse specialist. Ann urged Carrie to seek consultation from the university medical school perinatologist who was an expert in diabetic care.

Carrie and her husband wanted the consultation, but they were afraid of "rocking the boat." Both felt vulnerable. They were concerned about the welfare of the mother and baby. The obstetrician diagnosed the etiology of Carrie's symptoms as "deep seated anxieties" related to the unplanned pregnancy. The CNMs, at the same time, counseled with Carrie concerning the impact of this high-risk pregnancy on her life. While Carrie and her spouse acknowledged that the pregnancy was stressful, both felt that there was more to the problem than stress.

At 32 weeks gestation, the fulminating, pathophysiological crisis emerged. Hypertension, glycosuria, and ketosis increased. Physical symptoms incapacitated Carrie, and she stopped working full time. Carrie felt something was terribly wrong, yet when she questioned her health team, she received subtle cues that they "knew best" and that perhaps her symptoms were a somatic response to stress. Carrie felt she had been labeled as a *"troublemaker."*

With the support of her colleague Ann and her spouse, Carrie insisted on a glucose tolerance test. After the test, Carrie assumed that the results were normal, since her obstetrician did not phone nor did he respond to Carrie's phone calls concerning the test. Symptoms persisted, yet Carrie tried to ignore them and "calm down" as advised by her caregivers. Ten days after the test, the obstetrician phoned Carrie and told her that to his surprise the test *was abnormal.* (The results had been placed on her chart, so he had not received them promptly, yet the CNM and Carrie had not pushed for the results because they did not want to show disrespect to the physician. None of them wanted to disturb the balance of power by "rocking the boat.")

Carrie was placed on a 2200 ADA (Diabetic) diet. She was strongly motivated to follow the diet correctly for the welfare of the baby as well as herself. She visited the dietitian twice, kept a food diary, and carefully maintained a schedule of diet control. During this time, the caregivers explained the plan of care, but showed aloofness and avoidance behaviors. Self-care measures of urine testing and blood pressure determinations were discouraged. The message was clear. Carrie was to leave the management of her case to the obstetrician and midwives.

At 35 weeks gestation, Carrie's symptoms increased. Again her colleague Ann urged her to seek a second opinion. Since Carrie feared being labeled a "crock" or even worse, risk antagonizing and perhaps losing her caregivers, Ann intervened and phoned the consultant. The consultant thought that the symptoms were suspicious and agreed to see Carrie if her obstetrician, midwife, *or* Carrie consulted him.

A much relieved Carrie called her midwife to tell her of this news, and was shocked when the CNM expressed anger at Carrie and the colleague for going over the midwife's head and not following "appropriate" channels.

The midwife's response caused total emotional shock for Carrie. She felt guilty, betrayed, professionally put down, and fearful. Yet, with her colleague Ann's support, she asked her obstetrician to consult the perinatologist. The OB coolly agreed. He admitted Carrie to the hospital hoping to lower her blood pressure and to determine whether she was, "following the diet correctly." He ignored Carrie's request to call in the consultant. During a 2-day hospital stay, her B/P decreased and ketosis disappeared, except following meals. It was determined that a slow insulin release following a meal resulted in Carrie's ketosis and glycosuria. At this time Carrie was diagnosed as a Class A Gestational Diabetic.

After this hospitalization, Carrie, her spouse, and her colleague showed respect by reassuring the CNM and OB concerning their roles. At the same time, the CNM and OB gave some recognition to the client's ability for self-care, and acknowledged the importance of the support given by the colleague. Both sides expressed relief that the pregnancy was at term. While diabetic symptoms remained present, hypertension did not resurface.

Carrie's membranes ruptured at 40 weeks but labor did not follow. After a 10-hour induction, she delivered an 8 lbs. 6 oz. baby boy without complications. The only "infant of diabetic mother" symptom present was that the baby was plethoric with a hemoglobin of 22 mgm. High neonatal hemoglobin levels are associated with maternal-diabetic ketosis. At 4 days postbirth, bilirubin levels rose and the newborn was readmitted to the hospital for phototherapy. An exchange transfusion was avoided when the bilirubin levels dropped. The baby was discharged home on the eighth day after birth.

After the initial postpartum physiologic adjustment, Carrie felt well again. She expressed relief that this crisis was resolved, that she was well, and her baby healthy.

ANALYSIS

Of the four self-care paradigms formulated from the theoretical constructs found in the meta-analysis, the case study illustrates two:

self-care valuing by both client and caretakers and self-care valuing by client with imposed self-care disbelief by caregivers. These paradigms are pictured in cell 1 and 2 of Figure 1. Early in the pregnancy, all subjects in the case study expressed self-care value beliefs. When high-risk pregnancy evolved and Carrie questioned the management of her pregnancy, a client and caregiver self-care disbelief developed. Because of their separate cultural reasoning about patient care, the professional health team saw their role as one of control. Carrie saw herself as team member in care. All four could be described as being in culture shock: they did not understand why the other was "acting that way."

Kinlein (1977) defines self-care as the "activities a person initiates and performs in her (sic) own behalf in order to maintain life, health, and well-being." The self-care actions of the client, however, were an affront to the health care team. Woolery (1983) asserts that the pregnant woman, as a self-care agent, is not only capable, but has responsibility for decision making and goal attainment. Woolery assumes that goal attainment (namely healthy baby/healthy mother) is directly related to knowledge of pregnancy, therapeutic self-care demands. Therapeutic self-care demands (Woolery, 1983; Orem, 1971) are those actions aimed at: (a) supporting and promotion of life processes and normal functioning; (b) maintenance of normal growth, development, and maturation; (c) prevention, control, and cure of disease processes; and (d) prevention or compensation for disability. Carrie's identified therapeutic self-care demands are

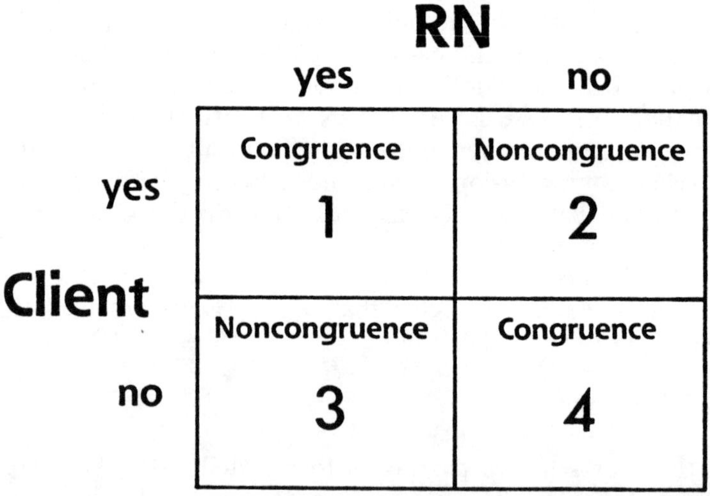

Figure 1. A model to guide self-care readiness.

parallel: (a) support and promotion of her own life and level of functioning as well as the fetus' during the threat of diabetes and pregnancy-induced hypertension; (b) maintenance of normal fetal growth, development, and maturation; (c) prevention or control of pregnancy-induced hypertension and ketosis; and (d) prevention of the "infant of diabetic mother" syndrome as well as noxious health outcomes for the mother. Yet, as this case study illustrates, in spite of her self-care knowledge (or perhaps because of it), the conceptual outcome was a self-care paradox. Instead of praising the client for her self-care initiative, the health team disapproved of her self-care behavior.

Power strategies between client and health team such as those seen in this case serve to erode utopian self-care practice ideology. In the end, the main self-care deficit for this client was identified as the professional health care system. That is, in order to abide by professional politics, that is maintaining the physician in charge pattern, the health caregivers became a barrier to self-care practice (Joseph, 1980; Marten, 1978).

The advocacy phone call placed by the colleague to the specialist, while termed inappropriate by the CNM, nevertheless provided a power base (in the form of a threat) for client, family, and colleague. This ultimately led to improved care and recognition of the client's self-care ability. Kohnke (1982) includes politics as a major proficiency needed by the advocate. In this case, politics served to return power both to the client and the health care team. That is to say, the client was given the opportunity to prove her self-care capabilities and likewise the health care team was afforded a measure of control to deal with the symptomatology once the client was correctly diagnosed. Therefore, the client verbalized satisfaction with the caregivers thereby *showing respect*. Once respect was shown, both the client, colleague, family, and CNMs demonstrated *cultural elasticity* by adjusting in spite of the culturally different behavior of the other. The obstetrician, however, remained an outsider to this adaptive self-care approach.

SELF-CARE PARADOX: A MODEL TO GUIDE
SELF-CARE READINESS

In our meta-analyses of the care study with the other studies, we developed self-care paradigms that indicate client and nurse readiness for self-care. The four paradigms seen in Figure 1 include paradigm 1, where client and nurse believe in self-care. We call this the *teamwork* paradigm. In paradigm 2 the client values self-care, while the nurse does not: the *troublemaker* refers to the label the nurse gives the client as they struggle for control. In paradigm 3 we see that the nurse values self-care while the client does not. The client in this paradigm is labeled *noncompliant*. In the remaining paradigm, both client and nurse agree that self-care is inappropriate. We call this paradigm *forced dependence*.

The factors influencing the formation of these paradigms center around the health culture value systems of nurse and client. When lay and professional cultures meet, they often have differing beliefs about self-care. We call these beliefs *cultural reasoning*. In Carrie's case, the differences in cultural reasoning were tied to self-care values. When faced with a possible client risk, the health team no longer felt comfortable allowing Carrie to participate in her care. In fact our data indicate that in the cultural reasoning of the health team their need to control was so strong that they were unable to assess Carrie's physical state properly. Even though they were supplied with a wealth of clinical evidence, dutifully reported by Carrie, they experienced what we call *cultural deafness* and *cultural blindness* so that their picture of Carrie was distorted. This is illustrated in Figure 2. When client and nurse have separate cultural reasoning, they experience culture shock, power struggles, fencing, and withdrawal.

Because the behavior of all persons in this case surprised the participants, they experienced culture shock. Carrie could not understand it when her professional colleagues began treating her, a maternity specialist, in what seemed to her a disdainful and cavalier manner. As the CNMs and the OB struggled with Carrie for control, they accused her of "playing doctor." Sick, afraid, shocked, and disillusioned, Carrie turned to what she saw as her only remaining source of help, her friend Ann. When Ann blew the whistle on the health team by calling the perinatologist, their culture shock heightened. The OB practiced fencing when he did not call in the consultant. The CNM tried to fence off her territory when she berated Carrie and Ann for "going over my head." Ann and Carrie used what we call the transcending variables to the self-care paradox, cultural reasoning and showing respect. They used cultural reasoning, working within the cultural framework of the other, when they called the

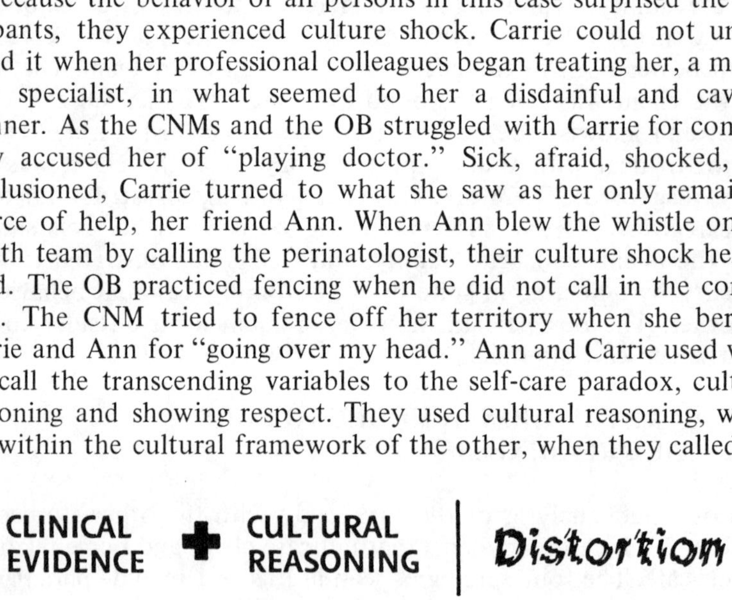

CLINICAL ➕ **CULTURAL** | Distortion
EVIDENCE   **REASONING**

Figure 2. Dynamics of the self-care paradox.

perinatologist. Knowing that the three professionals felt unsure in their new roles, they reasoned that threatening to expose their mismanagement was a greater risk for them than giving up some of their control to Carrie. This was a calculated political maneuver. It must be remembered here that Carrie's only demand was that they take care of her "response to actual or potential health problems" (American Nurses' Association, 1980, p. 9).

Carrie and Ann showed respect once the professionals went into professional action. When Carrie was finally hospitalized both she and Ann praised the professionals for their care. Positively reinforced, the professional team carried out their care quite well.

If we look at Figure 1 once more, we can see that when Carrie selected her professional health team she expected to spend her gestation and birth within paradigm 1; that is, she expected *teamwork* and she expected to be a team member. As she recognized the fact that the pregnancy was not going well, and asked her team to do the job she had hired them to do, they insisted by their reaction that they would not allow Carrie to tell them what to do. Carrie found herself an unwilling prisoner in cell two, the *troublemaker* paradigm. It was only when Carrie and Ann applied strategies of the variables cultural elasticity and showing respect that Carrie was able to break out of cell one to the comparative freedom of peace of mind and body found in paradigm 1, teamwork.

CONCLUSIONS

Self-care theory is an invention of the nursing profession, not the client. It is imperative that nurses, in their zeal to adopt a self-care approach, remember to assess the client's self-care value system. When self-care beliefs differ, strategies of *politics* and *showing respect,* as shown in the case of Carrie, can promote healthy outcomes for the client and for the nurse.

REFERENCES

American Nurses' Association (1980). *Nursing a social policy statement.* Kansas City: Author. (NP-63 35M 12/80).

Barnard, K. (1983). The case study method: A research tool. *American Journal of Maternal-Child Nursing, 8*(1), 36.

Brocato, C. (1982). *Right and left brain nursing: Pain assessment on an orthopedic ward.* Unpublished master's thesis, Northwestern State University, College of Nursing, Shreveport, LA.

Dickson, G., & Lee-Villasenor, H. (1982). Nursing theory and practice: A self-care approach. *Advances in Nursing Science,* October, 29–40.

Glaser, B. (1978). *Theoretical sensitivity.* Mill Valley, CA: Sociology Press.

Glaser, B., & Strauss, A. (1967). *The discovery of grounded theory.* Chicago: Aldine.

Harris, C. (1982). Circumcision: A cultural decision. In C. Uhl & J. Uhl (Eds.), *Proceedings of the Seventh Annual Transcultural Nursing Conference.* Salt Lake City: University of Utah Press.

Joseph, L. (1980). Self-care and the nursing process. *Nursing Clinics of North America, 15*(1), 131–143.

Kinlein, M. (1977). *Independent nursing practice with clients.* Philadelphia: Lippincott.

Kohnke, M. (1982). Advocacy—What is it? (1982). *Nursing and Health Care, 3*(6), 314–318.

Marten, L. (1978). Self-care nursing model for patients experiencing radical change in body image. *Journal of Obstetric, Gynecologic and Neonatal Nursing, 7*(6), 9–13.

Moore, P. (1982). *Response to menopause of selected northern Louisiana women.* Unpublished master's thesis, Northwestern State University, College of Nursing, Shreveport, LA.

Orem, D. (1971). *Nursing: Concepts of practice.* New York: McGraw-Hill.

Scott, M. (1982). *Childbearing beliefs of northern Louisiana Blacks.* Unpublished master's thesis. Northwestern State University, College of Nursing, Shreveport, LA.

Stern, P. (1980). Grounded theory methodology: Its uses and processes. *Image, 12*(1), 20–23.

Stern, P. (1983). Self-care from the patient's perspective: Issues of culture shock and control. Theoretical analysis. San Diego: Presented at the Society for Applied Anthropology.

Stern, P., Allen, M., & Moxley, P. (1982). The nurse as grounded theorist: History, process and uses. *Review Journal of Philosophy and Social Science 7*(1,2), 200–215.

Stern, P., Tilden, V., & Maxwell, E. (1980). Culturally-induced stress during childbearing: The Pilipino-American experience. *Issues in Health Care of Women, 2*(3–4), 67–81.

Woolery, L. (1983). Self-care for the obstetrical patient—A nursing framework. *Journal of Obstetric, Gynecologic, and Neonatal Nursing, 12*(1), 33–37.

TEACHING TRANSCULTURAL NURSING IN LOUISIANA
FROM THE GROUND UP:
STRATEGIES FOR HEIGHTENING STUDENT AWARENESS

Phyllis Noerager Stern, DNS, RN, FAAN
Dalhousie University School of Nursing, Halifax, Nova Scotia

Because of a dearth of material in the literature regarding the process of teaching transcultural nursing, it was necessary to do an analysis of processes, or feasibility study while at the same time engaging in the process of teaching transcultural nursing. Findings from this analysis indicate that a number of strategies can be used to help nurses integrate culturally sensitive material, but that the most important of these may be experiential learning.

FOREWORD

When I moved from the San Francisco Bay Area in 1980 to take a position at Northwestern State University in Shreveport, Louisiana, my agenda included teaching transcultural nursing. The process of working transcultural nursing into courses of study and public performance was both facilitated and at times precipitated by my own liberal West to conservative South transition. The teaching of transcultural concepts can present an interesting challenge regardless of what regional biases and traditions one may encounter. For those of you who appreciate the challenge, but lack the experiential frame of reference, I offer an autobiographical strategical review that you may find beneficial in implementing your own curricula. For those of you who have established your own strategies, your consensual validation affirms my effort, toward explaining the processes to the unfamiliar.

John Dillard, a specialist in Black English, explains that the verb

This was written when the author was Professor and Coordinator of Graduate Studies in Maternal Child and Family Nursing, Northwestern State University, School of Nursing, Shreveport, Louisiana. This paper first appeared in J. Uhl (Ed.), *Proceedings of the Eighth Annual Transcultural Nursing Conference.* Salt Lake City: University of Utah Press, 1983.

"to be" connotes a useful time-span dimension of considerable extension and contraction (1981). Thus the statement "I trying" means
that I am trying right now. "I be trying" on the other hand, tells you
that I have been trying, I am trying right now, and I am likely to go
on trying. Because so little has been written about the process of
teaching transcultural nursing, I have treated the experience as a
piece of inductive research, that is, I gathered data, attempted to
order it into patterns related to the real world, and applied the findings to the study population for their assessment of relevance and fit.
In sum, one could say that as a teacher of transcultural nursing,
"I be trying."

NURSE-TEACHER AS RESEARCH INSTRUMENT

Before designing a formal course of studies in transcultural nursing, strategies for teaching the discipline were tried out on a number of audiences, primarily students and attendees at professional
meetings. One might say this constituted a process-of-analyzing
process. Because of a dearth of methodology papers in the literature
that deal with the process of teaching transcultural nursing, this
study can be viewed as one of feasibility. Even though Uhl (1980)
provides a notable and useful work, it is not accessible to computer
search.

QUESTIONS

This research addressed the following questions: (a) how can
students in bachelor of science in nursing (BSN), and master of
science in nursing (MSN) programs, located in a conservative southern community be helped to gain heightened awareness regarding
culturally sensitive issues? (b) How can these students be helped to
incorporate cultural sensitivity into their practice?

Background

As I thought about teaching transcultural nursing, I referred to
the Chater (1975) framework for curriculum development. That
is, I knew I would have to take into account the setting, the students,
and the subject involved in any course of studies I might attempt.
The setting and the students are the main focus of this paper. The
subject is described in transcultural, anthropological, and other
literature.

Content

Content for my transcultural teaching evolved from the anthropological literature, the now quite respectable volume of transcultural nursing literature, from my own work, and from the experiences of students.

In general, authors whose work appears in the transcultural nursing or anthropological literature, stress the importance of heightening student awareness to the value systems of other cultures. Several authors point out the relevance that knowledge of these values has for nursing (Osborne, 1968; Leininger, 1970; Brink, 1976).

Generally, authors in the two disciplines suggest field study as essential to student learning. Several authors have described mass field studies where a whole class of students moved to another country for a time. Bond (1981), for example, reported taking students to Mexico. Richardson (1979) describes a comparative study of health care systems in England and Atlanta, Georgia, that involved an interdisciplinary group representing medicine, nursing, and sociology. Budgetary constraints prohibited us from undertaking such a large scale field study, however it was nevertheless utilized within the region.

Process

Dennis (1982) uses a multimedia approach for an introductory anthropology course. Borrowing an idea from Hogg of the University of Oregon (1974), Dennis runs a film, with the sound turned off, of anthropologists in the field. Flanking this silent film are projected slides of people from various cultures caught in the act of performing the activities of daily living. To his visual display, he adds tape recordings of the music of West African natives, native American tribes, and a selection from Johann Sebastian Bach. Taking a lead from Dennis, I used one or two sequences of "Cultural Diversity of Nursing Practice,"* a slidetape series on cross-cultural nursing.

I found Chrisman's (1981) paper, "Anthropology in Nursing Education" to be particularly helpful for the fledgling professor attempting to teach transcultural nursing for the first time. His paper stands alone as one in which the author discusses both the

---

*For further information contact: Concept Media, P.O. Box 19542, Irvine, CA 92714.

theoretical perspectives such a course of studies might take, and ways of getting the point across. He also shares the problems he encountered teaching BSN and MSN students. The element of Chrisman's teaching style that I admired the most, was his effort to learn more about nursing in order to make his course relevant. He showed us evidence of this knowledge by citing nursing authors in his papers. As he learned from his audience, a sense of respect for that audience evolved. This process carries through to patient teaching. For example, Pam Brink (1981) once said to me, "What's all this stuff about patient teaching? We should be learning from the patient!"

I learned from my audience as I progressed through my study-lectures, and seminars became data collecting devices. I took careful notes on how students and other audiences reacted to *what* I said, and *how* I said it. This clarified differences and similarities in points of view between me and members of the audience. Curriculum evaluators might call this responsive investigation (Guba & Lincoln, 1982). In other words, one responds to one's audience: what they want to know, what their concerns are, and what the issues are. These audience concerns guide investigation.

Change

Articles taken from the many works on planned change provided a framework for my teaching plans. A piece by Afaf Meleis (1979) on developing a conceptually-based nursing curriculum in Kuwait described the use of a faculty core group to help implement change. I used a core group of faculty and students to help me present material about the values and beliefs of various cultures.

METHOD

Data for this study were collected over a 24-month period from August 25, 1980 through August 28, 1982. Subjects were professionals, clients, and students living in Louisiana. Data were analyzed using the constant comparative method of grounded theory (Glaser & Strauss, 1967). The experienced field researcher will find my process of data collection familiar. The substitution of audience for single informants or small groups however, may represent a departure from the norm.

Setting

Most of the fieldwork (lectures, seminars, and other data collecting devices) was limited to Shreveport, Louisiana, and its neighboring community, Bossier City. Shreveport, a community of 205,342 persons (Shreveport, Louisiana Chamber of Commerce, personal communication, August 21, 1982) is situated in the northwest corner of Louisiana. One of the things I find most remarkable about Shreveport is the stability of its population, "people stay on here for generations" (Stern & Cousins, 1982). Although the people of Shreveport tell me that racial integration has steadily increased over the past 20 years, I find black and white persons to be more segregated than I was accustomed to in California.

Barksdale Air Force Base is located in Bossier City, population 50,817 (Bossier City, Louisiana Chamber of Commerce, personal communication, August 30, 1982). Because airforce personnel and their families tend to move from place to place, all this coming and going, in comparison with Shreveport, lends a certain cosmopolitan air to the city. People with roots in all parts of the country live there. It is interesting to note that for whatever reason, Bossier City's public schools, in contrast with Shreveport's, are fully integrated. It is also of interest that private schools are much more prevalent in Shreveport than they are in Bossier City, owing perhaps to a variance in economic factors.

Students and Other Audiences

The undergraduate student population for this study were those attending a course in humanities and health care. Graduate students were enrolled in courses in maternal-child and family nursing, theories of nursing, and grounded theory. The total student populations was 354 persons. Additional data came from student clinical logs, papers, interviews, and course evaluations.

The response, concerns, issues, and needs of other audiences that were used as data were gathered from those attending professional meetings in Louisiana including those from the Nurses Association of The American College of Obstetricians and Gynecologists district meeting (1980), the Regional Perinatal Nursing Conference (1981), Louisiana School of Nurses Convention (1981), Louisiana Nurses Association State Convention (1981), Beta Chi Chapter, Sigma Theta Tau meeting (1981), and the Louisiana State University Medical School National Perinatal Conference (1981). The total audience for all groups neared 1,000 persons.

Faculty

Faculty involved in the data collection included colleagues at Northwestern, and graduate students from maternal-child and family classes. I functioned as general organizer and sometimes speaker.

Analysis

Data were analyzed using grounded theory methodology (Glaser & Strauss, 1967; Glaser, 1978; Stern, Moxley, & Allen, 1982). Grounded theory has its roots in symbolic interactionism. This point of view posits that persons have interchanges with one another on the basis of the meanings certain symbols have for them, and the ways in which they value these meanings. An example of how audience response was used as data follows. To me, the concepts of transcultural nursing seem worth passing on. Therefore, when I talk about these concepts, I watch my audience for reactions (body language, verbal response) that I then try to interpret. On the basis of these reactions, I modify my actions and the content I present. A nod then, gives me the impression that I made a point clear, a blank look indicates to me that I need to explain, or give an illustration that will have meaning for that student, and a deep frown or a clutched breast, suggests to me that I may have come on too strong. Like any astute researcher (or teacher), in order to clarify the reactions, I stop and ask the audience about them.

FINDINGS

Trajectory

Being sensitive to any xenophobic feelings the citizens of Louisiana might have toward me, and given my own xenophobia concerning citizens from a segregated southern community, my teaching of transcultural nursing continued through three clearly definable phases beginning with phase one, testing the water.

Testing the Water
I began safely by talking about Filipino health care belief systems. I moved on to some black folk health remedies I had heard about. I suggested that since no one has conducted studies concerning the efficacy of these traditional care prescriptions, criticism is not justified.

Making a Splash

After a year of sidling up to the subject, I summoned up my courage and plunged into the transcultural nursing proper. I had learned to trust myself, and my audience. During this phase I organized my cadre of guest speakers and got on with it.

Heading for Shore

Ongoing analysis of the data indicated that culturally sensitive care is a concept as acceptable to the citizens of Shreveport as it is to persons living in any other part of the country. The work done by my colleagues and myself in teaching concepts and awareness of transcultural nursing was something I felt I could look on as a successful venture.

STRATEGIES FOR TEACHING TRANSCULTURAL NURSING: SHOWING RESPECT

Successful strategies for teaching transcultural nursing discovered in this study can be roughly grouped under the theoretical construct, *showing respect.* Respect includes honoring one's audience and their beliefs, be that a client, colleague, or student audience. The categories that belong under this theoretical construct include modeling, using resources, and experiential learning. Incidentally providing reading materials proved more successful for graduate students than undergraduates. Therefore this strategy cannot be considered universally successful for this subject group.

Modeling

Students need an example from which they can learn. Modeling is a time-honored teaching strategy that is common to all cultures (Maxwell, 1979). A professor acting as model for transcultural nursing shows respect for the values and beliefs of clients, *and* of the student population. Data from this study clearly indicate that "professor attitude" had the strongest impact on student response to client beliefs. This comment from the data was typical, "I remember learning facts in nursing school—Jews don't eat certain foods, Catholics want final unction, but so what, you know—they were just facts. It's your attitude that made me care about what people believe in."

Using Resources

I was fortunate in having people resources at hand. Mary Scott, a graduate student, presented lectures on being the different one in a group (Scott, 1981). Pauline Mella, a graduate student from East Africa talked to students about health care in Tanzania (Mella, 1981). Trudy Dowden, another graduate student gave findings from her study of Vietnamese clients (Dowden, 1981), and my colleague, Chandice Harris (1981) presented the findings from her study of cultural decision-making and circumcision. One of the professors in languages at Northwestern chose Black English as an area for study. He presented the special syntax, uses of the verb "to be," and double and triple positives and negatives, all of which differ from standard English. Students joined in spirited discussions following these presentations. In addition to people resources, students reported that the cross cultural slidetapes were helpful to their learning.

Experiential Learning: Personal is Universal

In an effort to help students understand the meanings and values of transcultural nursing, I attempted to relate material to the experiential here and now—the here being Shreveport, the now meaning something they could feel in the classroom and that they could call back later. (To call upon Black English once more, something "they *be* feeling.") For example, to illustrate the danger of generalization I would ask, "how do you feel when I make a statement such as 'southerners feel' or 'southerners think'?"

At about this time, I presented findings in Seattle from a study I started when I moved to Louisiana, "Overcoming the Culture Shock of West Coast to Northern Louisiana Relocation" (Stern & Cousins, 1982). The paper described a participant observation study that indicated the differences between the two cultures of California and Northern Louisiana, and showed some problems in adjustment. The paper attempted to demonstrate the relationship between the culture shock of relocation, and the culture shock patients feel when they move into the strange and unusual world of health care.

I felt the points I made in the culture shock paper were valid. However, I must admit that I used a heavy dose of humor when I wanted to highlight cultural differences between San Francisco and Shreveport. This was all very well and good in Seattle, but when I was asked to present the paper back home in Shreveport, I began to think about the sensitive nature of southerners, and I was afraid my new friends might be insulted by what I had written rather than amused.

Some people were insulted, but surprisingly, more of my audience responded to what I had to say as a recognition of their own experiences in feeling culture shock. The most succinct comment perhaps, was from one young student who said, "You know, you're a culture shock to us too."

The paper on the culture shock of moving from San Francisco to Shreveport produced an emotional response of two kinds. First of all, natives of the area were surprised to learn that they could be thought of as "different." They were surprised too, to learn that another area of the country could be so different from Shreveport. "It sounds," wrote one student, "like life is too fast paced in California to enjoy the things in life which I consider important." A different sort of response came from members of the audience who themselves had suffered culture shock. Persons who had been through it were eager to tell of their experiences. One BSN student from a small country town east of Shreveport told us about a woman from elsewhere whom she found to be very different. "She was from up North—or was it Russia?"

We tried role playing in class. Students played the roles of clients with folk health belief systems and caregivers to those clients. This helped students work with two belief systems, their own and the client's (Scott, 1982).

Students also did cross-cultural interviewing. Undergraduate students were given an interview guide and asked to interview someone from another culture. Many students had trouble identifying their own culture, claiming to be "plain old American." Some students settled for interviewing subjects from another state, while others crossed ethnic lines of country or color. Students both enjoyed the experience and submitted creditable data.

We played "The Culture Game."[*] This game designed by Noesjirwan and Freestone (1979) simulates culture shock for the players. Participants play out the rules of two separate cultures, and then begin visiting back and forth without having the other culture's rules explained to them. Students reported feeling disoriented, frustrated, angry, and "paranoid" in discussions following the game.

I asked students for their help. Asking for help seems to me to be a useful strategy for allowing students to participate in the professor's work, and at the same time, experiencing mutual respect. Students helped me delete words and phrases offensive to southerners from the original version of the cultural shock paper, and they helped me to write this paper. I also asked students to help me design

---

[*]For further information contact: Kimbarra Educational Services P/L. P.O. Box 25, Hampton, Victoria, Australia 3188.

course material, and to provide an on-going critique of what we were doing. Thus courses of study became grounded in the data derived from student input. This method has been used by teachers for generations. I am simply attaching a new name to the process: grounded theory.

Outcomes

I was one of three professors assigned to the baccalaureate program for one nonclinical course. Therefore, I had no way to measure the effect transcultural nursing material had on the practice of undergraduate students. Graduate students, on the other hand, submitted clinical logs and papers that demonstrated increased sensitivity to other ethnic health beliefs. Students learned to *hear* their client's expressed needs. Said one, "I can hear my clients and they can hear me." They became more culturally aware, and they acknowledged that awareness. "Now I can acknowledge a black person's blackness," said one man, "before, I used to pretend it wasn't there."

CONCLUSION

The postulate that all cultural beliefs regarding the wellness-illness continuum merit respect represents the value system of transcultural nursing. Attracting disciples to this value system requires energy, ingenuity, and a strong faith that the audience can be converted to what the transcultural nurse sees as "the truth."

REFERENCES

Bond, M. L. (1981). A comparative analysis of two cultures—Considerations for nursing: One teaching methodology. In P. Morley (Ed.), *Published Proceeding of the Sixth National Transcultural Nursing Conference.* Salt Lake City: University of Utah Press.

Brink, P. J. (1976). *Transcultural nursing.* Englewood Cliffs, NJ: Prentice-Hall.

Chater, S. S. (1975). A conceptual framework for curriculum development. *Nursing Outlook, 23*(7), 428–433.

Chrisman, N. J. (1981). Anthropology in nursing education. In P. Morley (Ed.), *Published Proceedings of the Sixth National Transcultural Nursing Conference.* Salt Lake City: University of Utah Press.

Dennis, P. A. (1982). Introductory cultural anthropology: A multimedia presentation. *Improving College and University Teaching, 30*(2), 63–66.

Dillard, J. (1981, November). *Black English.* Lecture presented to Humanities 401, Northwestern State University of Louisiana College of Nursing.

Dowden, G. (1981, November). *Caring beliefs of Vietnamese clients.* Lecture presented to Humanities 401, Northwestern State University of Louisiana College of Nursing.

Glaser, B. G. (1978). *Theoretical sensitivity*. Mill Valley, CA: Sociology Press.

Glaser, B., & Strauss, A. (1967). *The discovery of grounded theory*. Chicago: Aldine.

Guba, G. G., & Lincoln, Y. S. (1982). *Effective evaluation: Improving the usefulness of evaluation results through responsive and naturalistic approaches.* San Francisco: Jossey-Bass.

Harris, C. C. (1981, November). *Circumcision: A cultural decision*. Lecture presented to Humanities 401, Northwestern State University of Louisiana College of Nursing.

Hogg, T. C. (1974). Untitled paper. Northwest Anthropological Conference, University of Oregon, Eugene.

Leininger, M. M. (1970). *Nursing and anthropology: Two worlds to blend*. New York: Wiley.

Maxwell, E. K. (1978/1979). Modeling life: A qualitative analysis of the dynamic relationship between elderly models and their proteges. (Doctoral dissertation, University of California San Francisco, 1979). *Dissertation Abstracts International, 39,* 7531A.

Meleis, A. I. (1979). The development of a conceptually based nursing curriculum: An international experiment. *Journal of Advanced Nursing, 4,* 659–671.

Mella, P. (1981, November). *Health care in Tanzenia East Africa*. Lecture presented to Humanities 401, Northwestern State University of Louisiana College of Nursing.

Noesjirwan, J., & Freestone, C. (1979). The culture game: A simulation of culture shock. *Simulation & Games, 10*(2), 189–206.

Osborne, O. H. (1969). Anthropology and nursing: Some common traditions and interests. *Nursing Research, 18*(3), 251–255.

Richardson, M. L. (1979). The potentials of cross cultural field study: Emory's comparative health care systems program in London. *Journal of Nursing Education, 18*(9), 46–52.

Scott, M. D. S. (1982, March). *Dealing with black childbearing beliefs in the clinical setting*. Seminar presented to Maternal-Child-Family Nursing II students, Northwestern State University College of Nursing, Shreveport, Louisiana.

Scott, M. D. S. (1981, November). *Awareness of cultural differences and similarities*. Lecture presented to Humanities 401, Northwestern State University College of Nursing, Shreveport, Louisiana.

Stern, P. N., & Cousins, M. E. B. (1982). Culture shock as a positive force: Surviving West Coast to Northern Louisiana relocation. In C. N. Uhl & J. Uhl (Eds.), *Proceedings of the Seventh Annual Transcultural Nursing Conference*. Salt Lake City: University of Utah Press, pp. 69–80.

Stern, P. N., Moxley, P. A., & Allen, L. M. (1982). The nurse as grounded theorist: History, processes and uses. *The Review of Journal of Philosophy and Social Science, 7*(142), 200–215.

Uhl, J. (1980). Implementation of components of transcultural concepts into undergraduate curriculum. In M. Leininger (Ed.), *Transcultural Nursing Care: Teaching, Practice and Research,* Proceedings of the Fifth Annual Transcultural Nursing Conference. Salt Lake City: Transcultural Nursing Society, 1980.

CONCLUSION

Phyllis Noerager Stern
Dalhousie University, Halifax, Nova Scotia

Understanding cultural reasoning enables the provider of care to sort out problems in casefinding, history taking, health teaching, compliance, client decision making, and in fact, all areas of care that involve interaction between caretaker and client. If you cannot get through to the client, and the client cannot get through to you, neither of you can get anywhere.

The concept of cultural reasoning is derived by comparing data from a number of studies that involved women and their families from various cultural groups. It might be well to mention here that some of these people resembled the caregivers in that they were from the same ethnic group. However, the problem of distorted communication between lay and professional persons still existed. (You do not have to look different to have different ideas.) These studies describe the way these women, or in some cases families, make decisions when they are well and when they are ill, what their parents taught them about how to take care of themselves, how they perceive their health care providers, and how those providers perceive them.

These studies of black, brown, yellow, and white women are meant to give the clinician some idea of the wide range of health values inherent in the study of cultural reasoning. These studies only begin to illuminate the mystery of why other people do not seem to internalize and act on our advice concerning health care.

INDEX